Retiring from medicine:
do you have what it takes?

Edited by
Harvey White

Foreword by
Sir Roger Bannister

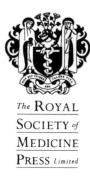

The ROYAL
SOCIETY of
MEDICINE
PRESS Limited

This book is published by the Royal Society of Medicine Press Ltd. The contributors are responsible for the content and for the views expressed, which are not necessarily those of the editor, of the Royal Society of Medicine, or of the Royal Society of Medicine Press Ltd.

British Library Cataloguing in Publication Data
A catalogue record for this book is available from the British Library
ISBN 1-85315-502-0

Cartoons by Phil Johnson
Phototypeset by Phoenix Photosetting, Chatham, Kent, UK
Printed in Great Britain by Ebenezer Baylis, Worcester, UK

Contents

Contributors

Editor

Ed – Harvey White is a consulting surgeon at the Royal Marsden Hospital and consultant surgeon at the King Edward VII Hospital (Sister Agnes). He is chairman of the Brendoncare Foundation for the elderly and chairman of the RSM Press. In addition to his work on medical committees he has written and edited articles in numerous surgical books and journals, including, most recently, contributions to *The Oxford Companion to Medicine*.

Authors

AKA – Aileen K Adams was a consultant anaesthetist at Addenbrooke's Hospital, Cambridge and lectured in the UK and Nigeria. She has always been a passionate traveller, both on professional business and whilst on leave. She enjoys out-of-the-way places and believes travel should be both a physical and an intellectual experience. After 18 years of retirement she feels she has learned a lot about adapting travel – and herself – to the inevitable problems of getting older each year.

AB – Alan Bailey has been chief medical advisor to Standard Life Healthcare, the private medical insurance division of Standard Life for the past eight years. Previously he was a director of BUPA Health Services where his work involved evaluating health screening and performing epidemiological studies on data collected at health check-ups.

GB – Gerald Bowden is a qualified barrister and chartered surveyor. He was active in politics and a member of parliament for Dulwich for over ten years between 1983–92. He currently practices specialised tribunal law and teaches law at Kingston University, Surrey.

JCB – John C Ballantyne is emeritus ENT surgeon at the Royal Free and King Edward VII Hospitals. He has been president of the Section of Otology at the Royal Society of Medicine and was made an Honorary Fellow in 1990. He has chaired the RSM Music Society and is late vice-chairman of the Retired Fellows' Society.

DB – Donald Birts is a director of Saunderson House Limited, independent financial advisers.

JPB – John Blandy is Emeritus Professor of Urology at the Royal London and St Peter's Hospitals. An addicted doodler, he illustrated his own textbooks and papers, and has painted and modelled his children. In retirement he continues to draw and paint from life at the London Sketch Club and to make portraits of his friends in bronze and oils. He is currently president of the Medical Art Society.

WRC – William R Cattell held several medical posts in Edinburgh and London before being appointed as a lecturer at St Batholomew's Hospital, London where he later established the NHS and academic departments of renal medicine. He became a senior physician and after retiring from the NHS in 1991 continued in private practice until 2000.

RC – Rex Chester spent 27 years in the paint and chemical industry and 28 years running the family estate in Hampshire. He was associated with the Grubb Institute of Behavioural Studies for over 40 years. In 1996 he founded a new charity, the *Students Exploring Marriage Trust*, designed to help young people gain a better understanding of the realities of marriage in the context of today's society.

KC – Kenneth Citron was a consultant respiratory physician at the Royal Brompton Hospital, London. He was an advisor to the Department of Health on tuberculosis and respiratory medicine and president of the British Thoracic Society. He is currently chairman of the Retired Fellows' Society of the Royal Society of Medicine.

ND – Neville Davis is a former vice-president of the Royal Society of Medicine. He was a general practitioner and is now a consultant occupational physician. He has been working at the medico-legal interface in his later years and recently co-authored *Medical Evidence: a handbook for doctors* published by RSM Press.

HF – Hazel French qualified as a solicitor in 1995 and currently works in the tax department of Fladgate Fielder. She specialises in wills, trust and estate administration, and tax planning for private individuals.

DH – David Hay served as medical officer in the Royal Navy Antarctic Guardship based in the Falkland Islands before returning to private practice in London. He was also chief medical officer for Commercial Union Assurance for 30 years. He has retired to a small farm in Hampshire where he grew up as a boy and has recently published *A flickering lamp; a history of the Sydenham Medical Club 1775–2000*.

MH – Mark Harries is a consultant physician at Northwick Park Hospital, Harrow, Middlesex and also clinical director (honorary) of the British Olympic Medical Centre. He has edited several sports medicine books including the *Oxford Textbook of Sports Medicine* and has been physician to six British Olympic teams since 1984.

SP – Susan Paine is the wife of a retired consultant, mother of four and grandmother of seven. She is the author of *Ever your Affectionate Florrie: letters from a Cavalier King Charles Spaniel to her two Mistresses* (1993) and has been a district commissioner of the Devon & Somerset Pony Club. She currently lives in Exmoor and retains a base in Oxfordshire.

EP – Elliot Philipp spent six years as a doctor with Bomber Command RAF before becoming a consultant gynaecologist after the war. In 1968 he moved to work as an infertility surgeon with Patrick Steptoe and Robert Edwards until the first test-tube baby was born in 1978. He continued to work as a surgeon and chaired an ethics committee concerned with infertility treatments. He has written several textbooks including *A History of Obstetrics & Gynaecology*.

PP – Peter Pilkington, Lord Pilkington of Oxenford, was an honorary canon of Canterbury Cathedral for fifteen years and is now canon emeritus. After ordination he was a curate for three years before embarking on an educational career, holding a succession of teaching posts ranging from schoolmaster to headmaster in schools such as Eton College, King's School Canterbury and St Paul's. He has also chaired the Broadcasting Complaints Commission and was a member of the parole board. He has been Education Front Bench spokesman and maintains an active role in the House of Lords.

BP – Brice Pitt is emeritus professor of psychiatry of old age at Imperial College, London and director of the Memory Clinic at the Hammersmith Hospital, London. He has an interest in the psychiatry of childbearing and is chair of the Association for Postnatal Illness. He has also been actively involved with the 'Defeat Depression' and 'Changing Minds' campaigns for the Royal College of Psychiatrists.

RS – Ron Staker has spent his entire career in healthcare management, commencing in the NHS in the 1970s, later moving into the private sector and owning his own nursing home company. For the past 10 years he has been chief executive of the Brendoncare Foundation, a registered charity based in Winchester caring for older people.

IS – Ian Snowley originally trained as a librarian. He joined the Royal Society of Medicine in June 1999 as director of information services. He is responsible for managing IT, library, and archive services for the Society's staff and members. Before joining the RSM he worked in the Department of Health as part of a team responsible for managing the roll-out of a new office automation system to 4,500 staff located in the London and regional offices.

PS – Penelope Steel has been involved with the Citizens' Advice Bureau service for 16 years, as a bureau manager, a specialist debt adviser and a volunteer. She is currently chairman of the South Region committee of the National Association of Citizens' Advice Bureaux.

JW – John Walton, Lord Walton of Detchant, was formerly professor of neurology and dean of medicine at the University of Newcastle upon Tyne before becoming warden of Green College, Oxford. He is a past president of the British Medical Association, the General Medical Council, the Royal Society of Medicine and the World Federation of Neurology. He has been a cross-bench independent life peer in the House of Lords since 1989.

DIW – Sir David Innes Williams was a urological surgeon at St Peter's Hospital, and later at the Hospital for Sick Children, Great Ormond Street. He has been director of the British Postgraduate Medical Federation and president of both the British Medical Association and the Royal Society of Medicine. He has also been vice-president of the Royal College of Surgeons and chairman of the Imperial Cancer Research Fund. He is now retired and has an active interest in medical history.

Foreword

Many doctors having completed some 40 years of service may be forgiven for the understandable feeling that they have earned a rest. Yet it is manifestly obvious that those who then re-engage in society around them are usually the happiest. There is a phrase sometimes used of the brain by neurologists, "use it or lose it". For retired doctors to throw themselves into new intellectual pursuits is almost second nature, as a lifetime of memories and experiences learnt from patients and colleagues arise unbidden. We now have the time to take on new challenges and discover the joy of new study, not for examinations but for fun – history, philosophy, art, music, writing – as this book shows so well. This applies equally to special skills using our hands to make new things through painting, sculpture and music. These skills were dormant or stifled or gifts we never knew we had.

Finally as a former sportsman you would expect me to stress the need for appropriate physical exercise – not the dash to the squash court with the risk of a ruptured Achilles tendon but whatever takes our fancy from gardening to walking the Fells or the golf course with appropriate companionship.

Whatever your ultimate choice from a dizzying variety of options, this excellent book will both guide you and inspire you, so you will, "Add life to years not just years to life".

Sir Roger Bannister

Preface

Now, of my threescore years and ten,
Twenty will not come again
And take from seventy springs a score,
It only leaves me fifty more.

From *A Shropshire Lad*
AE Houseman, 1887

These lines have been with me since my schooldays. Even as a young doctor, fifty springs seemed eternal and opportunities unlimited. Impending retirement now imposes an urgency on aspirations. There is a need to address priorities to ensure that the remaining time left does indeed become one of the most fulfilling periods of life. We must avoid looking back remorsefully on all those missed opportunities and the inevitable sadnesses that have overtaken one in the past.

In 1999 I decided to draw together the lectures from a course which I had developed for sixth-formers contemplating medicine and gather them together as a booklet, *A Career in Medicine: do you have what it takes?* This was well enough received to tempt me to do the same for those planning retirement. The obvious starting point was the Retired Fellows' Society of the Royal Society of Medicine which I conceived a few years ago and now has a large and active membership. The chairman and various members have made valuable contributions to this book. However, I have invited others to cover subjects which I felt should be included. There is some duplication between chapters but each can stand alone and may often be read separately. Contributions have been submitted willingly and with little need for alteration which has made my task as editor comparatively easy. This encourages me to think that the book is perceived as a worthwhile endeavour. As with everything we will have to work and plan if we are to achieve contentment and happiness in retirement. This little *vade mecum* is offered as a catalyst.

Some chapters are instructive, some have required great honesty and insight into emotional and private aspects of life. To all authors I am extremely grateful and hope that they will feel rewarded by the book being well received. I felt that most readers would be happy enough to make the politically correct gender adaptations where necessary in their own minds; if I have misjudged this I apologise.

Finally I must thank Mr Peter Richardson, managing director of the RSM Press and especially Miss Gabrielle Lowis, editorial assistant for their wisdom, encouragement, help and support.

Harvey White
London 2002

CHAPTER 1

The Retired Fellows' Society of the Royal Society of Medicine

R etirement is an opportunity. An opportunity to develop current interests, acquire new ones, to study, to travel and to spend more time with family and friends. For many people it provides the happiest and most satisfying years of their life. Yet some doctors do not adjust well to retirement, which they perceive as enforced idleness, loss of status and the gateway to old age. They think of retirement as "entering life's departure lounge in the hope that the flight will be delayed" (Nicholas Coni). Pessimism is supported by ageist jokes: "Growing old is like being increasingly penalised for a crime you haven't committed" (Anthony Powell); "I don't feel 80. In fact I don't feel anything till noon. Then it's time for my nap." (Bob Hope); "I'm at that age when just putting my cigar in its holder is a thrill" (George Burns). Wives traditionally complain about "twice as much husband on half as much money".

Recently retired doctors should be able to look forward to years of healthy, active and happy life. Having met many doctors in the Retired Fellows' Society, I am astounded at the breadth and vigour of their interests and activities and the very full lives they lead. I have learned that chronological age is not closely related to "growing old", "Growing old is no more than a bad habit which a busy man has no time to form" (Andre Maurios). Yet retirement is a rite of passage towards growing old, "Old age is the most unexpected of all things that happen to a man" (Leon Trotsky). However, it is something that needs to be anticipated and eventually welcomed, bearing in mind that growing old is usually better than the alternative. The gap that is left by retirement from a busy professional life can be filled by developing new interests and by meeting like-minded people.

The object of the Retired Fellows' Society is to give retired doctors and other people who have worked in all aspects of medicine, surgery, dentistry and veterinary medicine the opportunity to gather together and share their interests and enthusiasms, and study topics of medical and cultural significance. They are enabled to meet old friends and make new ones and help each other to get the best out of life.

The establishment of the Retired Fellows' Society

The creation of a group for retired Fellows in the Royal Society of Medicine was conceived in the hope and expectation that it would add to the quality of life of retired fellows by encouraging their continued participation in many and diverse activities. The Retired Fellows' Society was established in 1996. A committee was formed and a constitution adopted. Members of the committee were chosen for their known wide contacts and success in serving other organisations.

The difficulty in providing activities to satisfy members from such a wide spectrum of medical science was appreciated. Finding out about the interests of retired Fellows was the first priority. A survey of the 300 founder members showed that their average age was 72 years. A questionnaire about their interests revealed an astounding 280 different activities and preoccupations. Some were remarkably physical including cross-country skiing, swimming regattas, dinghy sailing, windsurfing, tennis and exercise programmes. Clearly these people are living life to the full. Personally I regard them as "OAPs" (Over Active Pensioners).

Many were keen to continue learning about advances in medicine and surgery. Music, theatre, history and the visual arts were popular. It was thought that, in addition, there might be a need that was not explicitly stated in the survey, namely the relief of loneliness. Retirement may cause loss of contact with friends many of whom have been professional colleagues. Loneliness may result from moving to a new and unfamiliar location on retirement. Most grave is the isolation caused by the death of a spouse or partner. It was therefore thought that a major objective of the Society should be to provide good opportunities for social gatherings in association with the meetings and other activities.

Fellows of the Royal Society of Medicine are particularly fortunate in having a gracious building well suited to their needs. The entrance hall is spacious and, in spite of its proximity to the crowds on Oxford Street, a tranquil place for meeting friends. The restaurant is elegant and there is also a buffet and bar overlooking a plant-filled conservatory. There is a quiet common room where Fellows can read current newspapers and magazines whilst seated in comfortable armchairs conducive to post-prandial somnolence. Throughout the building are portraits of famous people in medicine, which effectively reflect the history of British medicine during the last two centuries. The excellence of these club facilities helps in the task of attracting retired Fellows back to participate in the life of the Royal Society of Medicine. In addition the Society's famous Library has attracted many Fellows who during retirement continue medical reading or bibliographical research. However, such facilities and luxuries are not a pre-requisite for a group of retired doctors to flourish and attain fulfilment.

What the Retired Fellows' Society provides

Intramural Events

A selection from lectures, already given or proposed, gives a picture of the broad scope of the programme. These include the rise and fall of modern medicine, medical fraud hunters, the impact of law on medicine, and the proposed revalidation of retired doctors by the General Medical Council. All are areas in which profound and controversial changes have occurred during the professional lifetime of many Fellows. Lectures about tuberculosis in the 21st century, prostate cancer, sports medicine, travel medicine, advances in geriatrics, the pharmacology and therapeutics of maturity, and human reproduction have kept us in touch with medical advances.

Whilst some retired Fellows are remarkably fit and physically active, others are concerned about their own health during the ageing process and some events have been focused on healthy lifestyles and prophylactic medications in the elderly. "In this world nothing can be said to be certain, except death and taxes" (Benjamin Franklin). Hence the popularity of sessions on financial planning in retirement.

Lectures on medical history have generated much interest. Titles have included art, music and medicine, medical heroes, the history of gout, and illness in art and artists. Many Fellows have musical tastes and have enjoyed talks on Mozart and medicine, Elgar, and neuro-psychiatric aspects of music. Fellows, despite being retired, like continuing to hear and meet celebrated medical icons, both those who have been past pioneers as well as those currently in the spotlight. We enjoy the excitement of being at the cutting edge of major developments in medical science even though we are only spectators. Perhaps because of our long experience in the profession we may have something to contribute to help solve the ethical problems that can arise as a result of expanding medical horizons. We have been fascinated to hear Lord Walton of Detchant speak about his life and times and Lord Robert Winston describe the challenging discoveries in human reproduction. Some of the lecturers have been invited simply for their entertainment value but have been no less appreciated, such as the author Colin Dexter talking very amusingly about his life and his *Inspector Morse* books.

Luncheon is an important feature of the meetings. Long, leisurely, seated and with wine for those who wish it, it gives Fellows, their spouses and guests time to meet friends and make new ones – and important social objective for this group of retired people. We are fortunate that the Royal Society of Medicine provides excellent catering facilities, which are available for these occasions.

Extramural events

Extramural events are extremely popular and get Fellows and their guests out and about, may broaden their interests, and take them to places which they may not have thought of visiting, or which are not usually open to public view. Skilled guides are assured. Some visits are principally of medical interest, for example the medical equipment section of the Science Museum in London, others are of historical interest, including stately homes, or simply for their beauty, such as Mapledurham Watermill. Memorable visits include:

● A visit to the Royal Botanic Gardens at Kew included a lecture by a professor of botany, lunch and a guided tour with special reference to medicinal plants. Afterwards there was a tea, during which the conversation tended to be about the inspiration the guests had received likely to lead to improvements in their own gardens.

- At the Royal Army Medical College at Millbank, there was a talk by a Major General on the history of military surgery followed by lunch in the splendour of the officers' dining hall. Many of the visiting Fellows had poignant memories of when, as young doctors, they had received training in military medicine and surgery in these magnificent buildings. We were reminded that the establishment of this college was due to the inspiration and zeal of Florence Nightingale. Our visit was the last to be made before the place was closed as a military establishment and so marked the end of an era.

- A walk around Soho, notable for its multinational restaurants and its sex shops, would not be thought to be of much medical interest. However, we learnt that the area was home to Lady Mary Montague, pioneer of smallpox vaccination. Soho was also the site of the famous Anatomy and Medical School run by William and John Hunter and the first Hospital for the Ear, Nose and Throat in London. Frith Street housed Dr John Snow where he gave anaesthesia with ether for the first time in UK and whose observations of cholera in Broad Street in 1854 were the first to prove that it was a waterborne infection.

- Visits have also been made to the Institute of Naval Medicine, the ships *The Mary Rose* and *The Victory*, the Royal Veterinary College, the Speaker's House in the Palace of Westminster, and the British Library.

- Visits to theatre matinees have satisfied many tastes, both for the classics and for light entertainment, and have the added bonus that people may meet for lunch before the show.

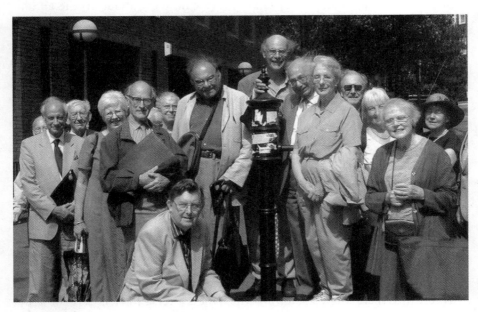

Figure 1 Retired Fellows by the Broad Street pump in Soho

The Annual General Meeting of the Retired Fellows is an opportunity for Fellows to make requests, and members of the committee are also available at the various events to receive suggestions. The great amount of work involved in arranging our many activities would not have been possible without the assistance of staff from the Academic Department of the Royal Society of Medicine.

The newsletter of the Retired Fellows' Society

The newsletter plays an important part in the life of the Retired Fellows. There are many original contributions on a wide variety of subjects, some of which are both intriguing and humorous. Topics have included wartime experiences, medical practice before the National Health Service, memorable patients, amusing incidents and anecdotes, philosophical meditations and poetry. I have been impressed by the high quality of some of the writing. Could we have an undiscovered Somerset Maugham out there? Fellows share their enthusiasm for hobbies and activities, for example, travel, photography, bird watching, music, art and historical research. They encourage others who are hesitant about acquiring new skills, for example, computing, providing a source of information and support. The newsletter provides a forum for letters and opinion and it contains regular reviews of books and medical literature likely to be of interest to the Fellows. Two special supplements have been published, one about tuberculosis and the other about doctors who have been notable both in medicine and in other fields.

Conclusions

The Retired Fellows' Society is popular and thriving. I have been astounded by the enthusiasm with which members have taken up new non-medical activities. Membership is 500 and growing. I believe it does so because it is designed to fulfil an important need for those who have retired from medical and allied professions, and it has succeeded in giving pleasure to many people. Retirement is an opportunity for a good life. Other professional organisations might do well to consider how they can improve the lives of their retired colleagues, and contemplate forming a group for retired people along the lines of the Retired Fellows' Society of the Royal Society of Medicine.

KC

Further information

For enquiries about the Retired Fellows' Society at the Royal Society of Medicine, please contact 1 Wimpole Street, London W1G 0AE; telephone: 020 7290 3948; website: www.rsm.ac.uk

CHAPTER 2

Family, friends and location

Location

Is the order of the title significant? Perhaps so, because surely location will depend on the first two, and their importance in your life. Retirement from the work you have done perhaps at the same centre for possibly the past 30 years must mean taking stock of where you live. You could be living in a now slightly over-large family house, bought way back at a very modest sum, compared with today's unreal values. You may feel that the general slog of keeping it up, and the wide spaces of the garden, are not entirely justified by the brief spells of full occupation when the family descend for Christmas or other gatherings. It is tempting to cash in, and make a move to something smaller, while blowing some of the gain on exotic travels. Your children probably struggling to rear and educate their own young may feel your priorities are wrong here. If you move, do you stay in the area, or do you want to site yourself where your passion for hill walking, fly fishing, small boat sailing etc. can be more conveniently enjoyed?

Beware of too radical relocation; surely as an intelligent professional you won't be led astray and make the classic mistake of burying yourself in a thatched cottage deep in Devonshire where you have never set foot before, and where you will die from either a heart attack or boredom within the year. There may be a region, be it the foothills of the Pyrenees or the Outer Hebrides, where you have often spent holidays and have promised yourself you will one day live. You are confident you have plenty of contacts there, are familiar with the locals and sure that friends and family will flock to visit you. Wonderful to escape the crowded roads together with the back-biting politics of your work place, and make a fresh start. Your ample spare time and wide experience of life means you can make a valuable contribution to your new community. Alas, the rural idyll is not and never was that simple. Reach below the happy veneer – the politics, the warfare, the trouble-makers are all there, and all the more intense because of the smaller number of participants. Be warned, at least be aware, if you choose this option.

Visitors will come, especially early on while you are comparatively fresh in their memory and they are curious to see how you are surviving. Your children will take a free holiday from you most years, but if you'd actually like to see them and their family more often, putting yourself at a significant distance is a mistake. They are probably at a particularly hectic stage in their careers, juggling work, children and social life; flogging down regularly during term time to see the grandparents will not come top of the agenda. Of course, you may not be able to stand your daughter-in-law, or the way she is bringing up your grandchildren, so may see this as desirable. But most of us do want to stay in touch, both with our children and our long established friends, those with whom we've shared the high and low spots of life. To do this, you need to be on hand, in my opinion to the extent of being at a reasonable distance for, say, Sunday lunch. For me, this means not much over an hour's drive. Distances may not be great in this country, but traffic is considerable.

Alternatively, one location where you could be certain of a steady stream of visitors would be central London – find a spot convenient for Harrods, or the West End, issue an open invitation, prepare a good stock of bed linen – your spare room will never be empty. This might have appeal for those who feel they've been long starved of culture in some remote fastness, and could now see shows, exhibitions, concerts etc. to their fill. The hefty price of London property might be a problem here, and the responsibility of accommodating teenage grandchildren thirsty for the bright lights of the big city could be worrying too.

Family

Retiring from medicine at 65 supposes you have been capable of doing a busy job up to that point, so you are unlikely to become decrepit overnight. Other chapters of this book deal with interests, culture and travel which you now have more time to enjoy. But for most of us, our family is the hub of life. One's children – unless they have developed into middle-aged hippies – are well past the agonised adolescent stage, and occupied with their own responsibilities. With luck they will have become quite tolerant of their aged parents, and will appreciate the time and support you can now give in small and larger ways. Being a reserve on the school run, attending the school play, even helping with the homework means you come to know your grandchildren well, and prepares the ground for taking over their household fairly effortlessly, so enabling the exhausted parents to have an occasional break alone. It is best to keep your criticisms of their offspring's food fads, untidiness, addiction to the computer/TV, choice of clothes and so forth, muted; a relaxed relationship is essential if there is to be useful and appreciated family inter-dependence. You can always let off steam to your friends, contemporary grandparents, and most will sympathise wholeheartedly. In return, you can rely on family labour to water your garden, feed the canary or even accommodate your dogs/cats when it's your turn to go on holiday. But this valuable and rewarding give-and-take is really only practical if you live relatively nearby.

Friends

Acquaintances can be many, but true friends are rarer. Those you were at school with, and have kept in touch over time, with whom you can always pick up where you left off, even if that was five or twenty years ago, are special. You are probably mutual god-parents, you will have been to each other's children's weddings, even parents' funerals, you may have shared a holiday house and remained on speaking terms. Such will always be a part of your life, even if you elect to live in Antarctica. But there will be others, also very good friends, perhaps former work colleagues, parents of children at the same school, neighbours you came to know well and with whom you found you had much in common. You risk losing touch with these if you move far away. Of course one hopes to continue to meet new and interesting people, and some of these you will come to know well and enjoy their company, but consider carefully before taking yourself to a place remote from easy contact with your long standing friends – you will miss them. It takes time and shared experiences of years to build true and relaxed familiarity.

Taking the plunge

Everyone's circumstances are different, there is no rule or guideline that will suit everyone. A move can be stimulating, a challenge, a chance to distribute or dispose of some of the clutter we all accumulate. The actual process may be pretty awful, but once the decisions of what to take, what to pass on to which child and what to throw out are made, and the unpacking is mostly done, it can be a lot of fun putting your imprint on a new house and garden. On average we are living longer; there is time to plant trees and see them grow to a reasonable size. But for most of us, I believe it is sensible to remain fairly close to the region where you brought up your family and spent most of your working life.

If you bought your added years, picked up a merit award or two, perhaps your yearning for places further off could be satisfied with a holiday property? You will have more time to visit and maintain this than during the busiest years of your professional life. Yet be mindful that all property can be a millstone, and make sure the pleasure such a refuge gives will sufficiently outweigh little local difficulties that may occur in your absence. That charming agent who undertook to deal with letting and maintenance on your behalf may melt away after your first year of ownership, leaving you prey to irate calls from the neighbours saying your cesspit is overflowing into their drive, or a noisy party of youngsters have been camping in your garden for a week and show no sign of leaving, do you know about them? If your retreat is in foreign parts, sorting out these happenings will be complicated by obstacles of distance, language and culture.

A move at retirement should not be necessarily thought of as your final change of address. Even if you toil on to 65 – and many now opt for an earlier departure – you can at least hope to have fifteen or twenty years of active life ahead. You may have been developing some interest, say a piece of research, a hobby or even a small business enterprise, with a view to giving it a real go when you say goodbye to the NHS, and you will head for a location that suits this. A few years pass, the deeply interesting results of your research have been expensively published at your own cost without making great waves, just a ripple in a small pond, or your passion for building and launching miniature rockets wanes, or you sell the small business – preferably at a fat profit. Now you may contemplate another move. It really isn't that difficult, and you will have had comparatively recent practice.

Most of us would choose to die in our boots rather than our bed, but this cannot be relied upon. As you creep or stride towards real old age, infirmities could be looming, so you may wish to scale down your surroundings physically, or site yourself nearer your favoured medical adviser and perhaps within reach of public transport. You may have eyed up and selected a care home should this become necessary, or take yourself to some courtyard development for senior citizens, where you could feel secure and more likely to retain a degree of independence for as long as possible. If the body is failing, the mind should be kept challenged: it could be important at this stage to be close to libraries and local colleges; classes for the 'third age' are increasingly popular, see the chapter in this book on *Lifelong learning* p39 for a detailed discussion.

It has to be your choice: you may want to carry on struggling with the weeds despite stiff joints, and the need to put on strong reading glasses to prune your roses or unblock the gutters. However, you may decide these challenges are no longer for you, and a shift to comparatively maintenance-free quarters should be made. At all costs remain adaptable: do not dismiss new technology as only for the young, master the damned video/PC/microwave, and consider a change of domicile as experimental. Good luck!

SP

CHAPTER 3

Marriage – a developing relationship in retirement

Don't talk of love – Show me!
Eliza Doolittle, *My Fair Lady*

When the Editor first approached me to ask if I would be prepared to write this chapter, I thought he must be joking, and was reluctant to take him seriously. How could it be sensible to ask someone who has had three failed marriages, to write a chapter on "marriage – a developing relationship in retirement"? Perhaps it is the fact that at the fourth attempt I am more happily married than I could possibly deserve, and have been so for the past six years. As my wife repeatedly tells people, "I am Rex's fourth and last wife". Perhaps it has something to do with the fact that five years ago I started what has become a new charity called the "Students Exploring Marriage Trust" which exists to help young people get a better understanding of the realities of marriage in the context of today's society.

What I feel the need to make quite clear at the outset is that I approach this task in the deepest humility, as someone whose track record in the marriage stakes has, until comparatively recently, been strewn with three catastrophic falls. In no way do I aspire to teach anyone anything, or to provide a recipe, or a set of guidelines, which, if adhered to, will automatically lead to a long and happy retirement. What follows are a few thoughts and reflections about the subject, coupled with one or two stories from my own experience which seem to me to illustrate points that may be worth thinking about. Perhaps in a way this in itself is one of the keys to retirement – it needs thinking about and not to be taken for granted as though nothing was going to change.

The institution of marriage – from whence does it come and what does it mean?

I could think of no better place to start than to go back to the beginning. For me, "the beginning" is to be found in the second chapter of Genesis where God offers his gift of marriage for all of mankind for all time.

> v.18   *it is not good that man should be alone; I will give him a helper as a partner.*

v.24   *therefore a man leaves his father and his mother and clings to his wife, and they become one flesh.*

Herein lies the perennial challenge of marriage – how to become, and to remain, "one flesh", yet at the same time, how to give freedom to each other so that both parties to the marriage are able to maintain their own identity, and to develop and grow as human beings.

This is spelt out in the Alternative Service Book (1980) under the heading "The purposes of marriage" (and I regard this not in terms of rules imposed by the Church but rather as the distillation of best human practice over many centuries). "Marriage is given that husband and wife may comfort and help each other, living faithfully together in need and in plenty, in sorrow, and in joy", and I guess one might add, "and in retirement"!

This seems to lead naturally into my first story which, for me, provides a brilliant and most moving illustration of what intimacy can mean in retirement. The incident happened in the waiting room of our local surgery. The parties concerned, Hilda and Len, both in their early eighties, had each lost their respective spouses through death in the past eighteen months. Hilda was sitting in the waiting room when Len walked in. Seeing Hilda he walked over to her and said, "do you mind if I sit next to you?" "Of course not" she said and Len sat down. Turning to Hilda with his eyes filling with tears, Len said, "Isn't it awful?" Hilda replied, "Yes Len, it is awful." Len then said, "Do you mind if I hold your hand?" With great understanding Hilda said, "No Len, of course not.", "You know," he said, "I miss that so much."

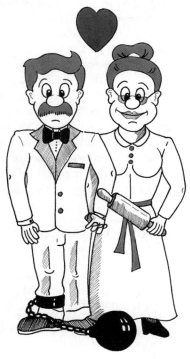

This is perhaps not quite the definition of intimacy that would occur naturally to the mind of a feisty teenager but as an illustration of what companionship can mean in old age it says it all.

Retiring from medicine today

Those who are retiring from medicine today will, rather like farmers, have seen their profession change out of all recognition and this will in itself have a huge bearing on their thoughts and feeling in the approach to retirement. What was very much an art form in which intuition played a significant part is now in danger of becoming too scientific. Yet, in terms of clinical success, those doctors who investigate less and write down less but rely on a deep-seated understanding of human nature and the human psyche, often have a significantly better record in curing patients than those who rely more heavily upon scientific wizardry.

Another dimension is the esteem in which the doctor is held by his patients and the public at large. In years gone by, the local GP was held in high regard within the community, someone who could act as a friend and confidant – as well as practitioner. Today, that position has changed dramatically. Doctors have become simply members of one enormous service industry, having to find larger and larger sums of money to fund their practices and to pay the premiums on their professional indemnity.

When retirement comes, a doctor may be emotionally and physically exhausted and have to integrate in a society where his pension and esteem are less than he might wish. A continuing happy marriage is, therefore, ever so important.

Choosing the moment to retire

The challenge imposed upon the marriage by retirement does not, of course, begin at the moment when the doctor leaves his surgery for the last time. The planning of when to retire is critical. The fact that retirement seems more threatening financially than it used to makes it more difficult to retire. In many ways, 65 is too late yet the NHS pension scheme is geared to retirement at 65 and financial penalties for early retirement are severe. In addition, many of those schemes that were sold to doctors on the basis that they would provide financial security in retirement have, rather like school fees insurance, fallen seriously short of expectations. So the financial downside of retiring at, say, 60 looks daunting. However I suspect that many doctors will decide to retire early partly because the nature of the job doesn't provide the satisfaction it used to.

How will you know when is the moment to retire? A GP I have known for many years suggested that the time to retire was when you start feeling nervous about the job. You become more aware of boredom and fatigue. Perhaps you give up doing nights and weekends and when you do this you begin to cease facing up to the challenge of medicine. This is a time when the marriage will be tested in an entirely new way. The doctor will need to share his thoughts and especially his feelings with his wife, and she will need to exercise all the understanding, the compassion and the love she can muster.

The late Sir Ronald Gibson, former chairman of the BMA, once said that "everyone needed an 18 month course to prepare for retirement". So choosing the time to retire must, if humanly possible, be taken as a joint decision if the retirement is to get off on the right foot with both parties feeling they have acted positively.

Retirement – a golden opportunity waiting to be grasped

I always remember asking my late father's chauffeur what retirement meant for him and his reply was, "Being able to have a lie-in and not feeling guilty about it". Retirement can be, and usually is, a very rewarding time. It provides much greater freedom than husband or wife will probably ever have known in their lives – freedom from responsibilities at work or raising children, freedom from routine, freedom to choose and to plan their lives. So long as health permits, there are great opportunities out there waiting to be grasped.

Perhaps that last word 'grasped' is critical because those opportunities will not just happen of their own accord, they have to be grasped, which means that there has to be a significant element of planning. Much will depend on how much each partner still seeks fulfilment and how far their circles of friends overlap. Do they have shared interests in, for example, the field of sport, gardening, historic buildings, fine arts, or just enjoy walking arm in arm?

A joint venture and the need for planning

It may seem to be a statement of the obvious – but then we human beings can be remarkably good at failing to notice the obvious – that retirement from medicine will invariably entail a huge adjustment. The doctor will have entered the profession with a sense of vocation and been involved with it for around 40 years. He is used to having an office, secretarial services, partners, a circle of professional friends, and has gained the respect of colleagues, nurses and others. More importantly, perhaps, he will have earned the gratitude of patients, some of whom have, in the course of time, become friends. Having been in a vocational occupation there will be the feeling of having done something worthwhile in life.

The discussion about retirement should start long before the appointed day, most particularly, as I have referred to earlier in the context of deciding when to retire. However, as with so many things in life, you can try to imagine and to anticipate for all you are worth but it is only when you are actually in the new situation that you can really begin to come to terms with reality. Because of the magnitude of the sea change retirement represents, I would suggests that it is marked by a major break in what has hitherto been the domestic routine. If the couple has always wanted to hike in the Swiss Alps, explore the Galapagos Islands, or bicycle across the United States of America, now is a great time to do it. Such a project will of itself take some planning, it will provide un-pressured time for talking and it will begin to create a new piece of shared experience to look back on and enjoy together.

I feel that it is not for me to list all the items that might feature on a planning agenda to be discussed during the course of such a break. Other chapters in this book will cover this. There do seem to me, however, to be two items that outweigh most others. The first is the importance of maintaining intellectual and mental stimulations as well as physical health and well-being. The second is the need to come to terms with the realities of ageing and acceptance of the inevitability of death.

The marriage relationship

I was amused to read the other day Fay Weldon's response to the question "had she got better at relationships as she had got older?" She replied, "Oh yes, you do learn. Your judgement about people refines itself, you begin to know what is going to happen next, you learn to hold your tongue, and you learn that things will wait a day". Somebody once said to me that there are as many different types of marriage as there are stars in the sky so there can be no question of a "one size fits all" approach. To say that "marriage is what you make it" sounds like a bland truism but nevertheless that is the case. Perhaps in retirement husband and wife need to learn to talk to each other in a new way, to listen to each other and not just to the words. I have always treasured that impassioned plea of Eliza Doolittle in *My Fair Lady* when she sings, "Don't talk of love – SHOW ME," because at the end of the day marriage is about love. Fine words are all very well but what Eliza was seeking from Professor Higgins was action.

I'd like to conclude this chapter by quoting from a *Thought for the Day* broadcast given by Elaine Storkey. She was responding to a proposition put forward by the much married pop star, Rod Stewart, that the words "till death us do part" should be removed from the traditional wedding ceremony with the marriage certificate reshaped along the lines of the old dog licence and renewed annually. He felt it was unrealistic in the 21st century to expect a couple to stay together for life.

Elaine Storkey responded, "It's not the contract which needs to be renewable, but the marriage; not an annual dog licence we need, but a daily sharing of intimacy time and good communication. Perhaps the real issue for the 21st century is an attitude problem. If we put self-fulfilment at the centre of all relationships, commitment is a chore and vulnerability a threat. And we can never fully recognise the God-given glory of that other person. To do that we need love and acceptance and a faithfulness which continues for better, for worse, till death parts us."

RC

CHAPTER 4

Medical screening and insurance

In theory, the idea of detecting a disease before it manifests itself clinically seems reasonable, particularly to the layman. In practice, we know it is fraught with difficulties. The medical profession in Britain is fairly cynical about the benefits of screening. Years ago fulfilment criteria were laid down before screening procedures were adopted in the NHS, these included the very obvious principle that the disease should be treatable and that treating it early made a difference to the prognosis. Subsequently very few adult screening tests have been shown to meet these criteria.

Despite this, for many years there has been encouragement in the USA for well people to submit to an annual physical examination. I have, for example, a pamphlet produced nearly 20 years ago advising the healthy middle-aged and older person to have, among other things, blood cholesterol checked regularly, the stools examined for occult blood, sigmoidoscopy every four years, and annual mammography for women. But the big question remains: what difference can we make to our prognosis by submitting ourselves to screening tests at regular intervals?

Coronary risk factors and screening

As the incidence of ischaemic heart disease (IHD) rose between the wars, there was a view that it could not be prevented. It was only in the 1960s, when the medical profession realised that cigarette smoking was related to IHD, that prevention became a realistic aim. At about the same time American studies suggested that blood pressure was related to stroke and IHD, and defined the relationship between a nation's coronary incidence and its mean blood cholesterol level.

A high proportion of the medical profession gave up cigarette smoking and doctors' IHD rates are today generally among the lowest in the country. But IHD remains the largest killer and disabler of middle-aged men. Blood pressure and high blood cholesterol levels can be effectively treated and, if reduced, improve the prognosis for IHD and stroke. Low density lipoprotein cholesterol is the important fraction of the total cholesterol and there are a number of effective drugs on the market that can reduce this. However, further benefit may be obtained by tackling the other factors which make up what has recently been defined as *metabolic syndrome* in which one or more of the following factors are present: obesity, high blood triglyceride level, hypertension and raised fasting blood glucose.

The resting electrocardiogram is an insensitive test for early IHD; an exercise test improves the detection rate but is more appropriately indicated for the elucidation of symptoms. More sophisticated non-invasive methods of imaging the coronary tree are available but have not taken off as screening tests. The backbone of prevention involves avoiding smoking, eating a healthy diet, maintaining an ideal weight and taking adequate exercise alongside treatment of the metabolic syndrome with appropriate drugs. These tests are carried out by technicians and need not involve a doctor. The interpretation, however, is a medical matter. An unhurried consultation gives time for discussing domestic and other stresses and interpreting the screening tests. It needs to be carried out by someone interested in this preventive approach who also keeps up-to-date with the science surrounding the subject.

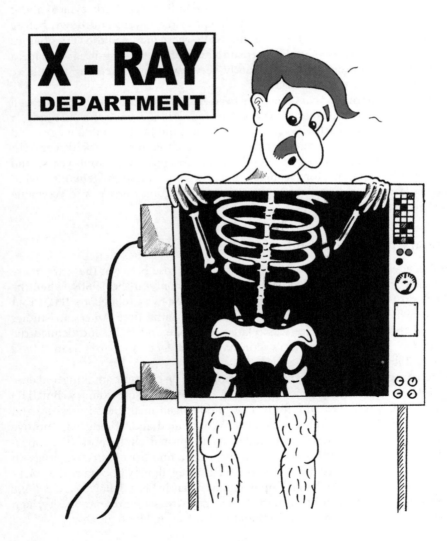

Cancer screening

This is a difficult time to give advice about screening for cancers. Scientists, economists and evangelists clash regularly over the value of screening for breast, colorectal and prostate cancer – diseases all common in the retired population. Tests for early detection are all available but the real question is "does early detection affect mortality?" Consider the following examples:

- Randomised studies of mammography screening suggest that this is effective and it has been available to women over 50 on the NHS for many years. Breast cancer mortality is declining but in all patient groups, not only in the screened group. However, recently published reviews have been critical of the different treatment received in the screened and control groups in the evaluation studies, suggesting that the screened group had received more aggressive treatment than the control group. So a definitive conclusion has yet to be reached.
- In the absence of a family history of polyposis, the question remains whether regular examination of the stool for occult blood (FOB) and colonoscopy follow-up for positive results really saves lives? After years of study, the results are again inconclusive.
- Prostate specific antigen (PSA) is a sensitive indicator of the presence of early prostate cancer. But there is little consensus on the treatment of early prostate cancer as it is thought that most people with prostate cancer die with it rather than from it.
- Cervical cancer screening is wise while sexually active and other gynaecological check-ups are recommended if one is receiving hormone replacement therapy.
- Screening for ovarian cancer is being evaluated.
- As malignant melanoma becomes more common, photographs of suspicious lesions may be taken and compared over time as a useful indicator of change.

These screening tests are available privately; the fact that they may not have been proven to save lives, by the rigorous criteria that have been set, does not necessarily mean that they are useless. This is the evangelist's view.

Effectiveness aside, the other problem for hard-pressed diagnostic facilities is sorting out the true positives from the false results. Screening tests are no more than a guidance to decide if more invasive investigations are worth employing. Biopsies, for example, frequently turn out not to confirm the histology that is being screened for. In a healthy population the incidence of the disease is so low that even tests which are highly sensitive have a low predictive value. Thus, the health economist takes the view that screening is not cost effective.

Screening and diagnostic tests are not without their own risks. The radiation risk of 30 years of mammography, the risk of gram-negative septicaemia after transrectal prostatic biopsy or bowel perforation during colonoscopy are examples. Certainly when mammography was started in New York in the late 1960s, the radiation used would be unacceptable nowadays; technology has improved and the present radiation risk is extremely low. Antibiotics are now routinely given to cover prostatic biopsy – something that used not to be the case – and perforation during colonoscopy in healthy patients is probably less than one in 10,000 in the best hands.

The side effects of treatment and the quality of life have to be considered in the risk benefit analysis. But these are day-to-day decisions that practitioners help their patients to make. What should they do for themselves? It is not always so easy to decide. And there is a further problem: in the private sector there are vested financial interests behind encouraging screening. There is profit in it, whereas in the NHS the opposite is true and the NHS can hardly cope with sick patients let alone the "worried-well".

Conclusions

The final decision regarding what screening tests the retiring practitioner decides to submit to will be a very personal one. It will take into account what I have said above. It should include a discussion with an experienced screening doctor who does not hold a vested interest in the system. One's attitude to life, one's family and past history, one's social habits and beliefs are all relevant in taking the decision. Personally I believe on a scientific basis that breast screening is likely to prove the most beneficial, faecal occult blood testing is no more than sensible in retirement and I would put the value of the PSA at the bottom of the list for now in the knowledge that research is aiming to produce a predictor for the type of prostatic cancer that benefits from treatment.

Finally, there are a number of day-to-day functions that cease to be efficient as we get older, not through disease but as a result of the normal ageing process. Regular hearing and vision checks can improve the quality of life and reduce accidents. Regular ophthalmoscopy and screening for glaucoma over the age of 60 (or the age of 55 if there is a family history) will detect conditions that can be halted or corrected. Detection of cataract early, for instance, allows one to join the NHS waiting list before it becomes necessary to stop driving.

One can see from these observations that the perceived wisdom and the science will continue to change. Most important of all is advice from a younger colleague with an interest (not financial) in this type of medicine.

Private medical insurance

It will be clear to any medical practitioner that, however well-intentioned successive governments are towards a fully comprehensive NHS, things will only get worse as the proportion of older people increases, putting more pressure on services, particularly for elective surgery and cancer treatment. At the same time, private medical insurance (PMI) premiums have risen spectacularly in the last ten years. PMI is a product that is relatively cheap when you're young, and you have little call for it, and can probably afford it. Insurance premiums go up with age and for people on a fairly fixed pension can take a large slice of their income.

PMI doesn't cover chronic conditions. After a stroke, for instance, the insurers will pay out for assessment and during early signs of recovery – but as soon as there appears to be a slowing up of progress it will be deemed chronic and cover will stop. But PMI should cover acute exacerbations of a chronic condition. For example, asthma may have periods of relatively inactivity contrasting with occasional acute exacerbations – the latter periods would be covered.

Most PMI won't cover pre-existing conditions on the principle that you can't insure your house after the fire has started. But the wording of the policy needs to be studied carefully. It usually states that it will not cover conditions for which the policy-holder has sought advice on the symptoms. So if the diagnosis changes after the policy has been effected, you might think this was a different condition – not so if the symptoms were present before the policy was taken out, even if they were ascribed to a different diagnosis. The method of establishing whether a condition is pre-existing varies. An underwritten policy requires applicants to answer a questionnaire concerning their past medical history. Any illness that is admitted, and its related conditions, will be excluded in a special clause in the policy.

Alternatively, the policy may be subject to a moratorium. This usually takes the form of excluding from benefit any condition that the applicant has suffered from in the previous five years, for the first two years of the policy, provided that the policy-holder has not received advice or taken treatment for that condition for a two-year period. Insulin-dependent diabetics would, therefore, be excluded for any diabetic problem forever.

An insurance policy is an annual contract. At the end of the year a new premium has to be paid and any money previously paid belongs to the insurers. In PMI there is, as yet, no premium loading as poor risks are subject to with life assurance. But several companies now offer "no-claim bonuses". Some insurers will not offer insurance to people over a certain age but SAGA policies, for example, have no age limit. Some insurers sell comprehensive policies for medical practitioners at a discounted premium, recognising the lower claims experience. As far as I know, you cannot nowadays send a case of wine to a colleague and claim off your health insurance.

So what is a sensible policy for the retired practitioner? Many colleagues will still treat other members of the medical profession for free, but private hospitals will always charge and charges vary. The cost of a hip replacement, including the

Table 1   The cost of common elective procedures
(Estimated from the claims database of Standard Life Healthcare)

	£
Angiography	1,500 – 2,000
Cataract	2,500 – 3,500
Coronary artery bypass graft	11,000 +
Hysterectomy for benign conditions	3,500 – 4,500
Hip replacement	6,000 – 8,000
Prostatic resection (transurethral)	3,000 – 4,000

surgeon and anaesthetist fees, may be up to £8,000 (see table 1) if there are no complications. Shopping around hospitals getting quotes can often reduce the charges for a self-payer and may may give you the option of a guaranteed price.

Today, policies with a high excess are available – this is the amount of money that the policy-holder pays before the insurer becomes liable. The higher the excess, the cheaper the policy: for example, a policy with an excess of £5,000 may cost one-third of a fully comprehensive one. If you can afford it, why not have high excess PMI and put the remainder of the premium into an ISA or similar tax efficient saving each year. The money you save can be used to pay for the smaller health bills (or use the NHS in areas where it is working well). In this way you have a greater say over what happens to your money and the reassurance that if the medical expenses go over the excess you are covered. But read the policy carefully and make sure you understand the conditions. All reputable PMI companies have a medical advisor who would be happy to talk to you on the different policies that might be suitable.

AB

CHAPTER 5

Fitness

Proof that exercise prolongs life is lacking, but what can be stated with reasonable certainty is that regular exercise prolongs an active life, and to that extent at least, is highly desirable. Fitness is a state that is reached after a process of adaptation to regular physical work, above and beyond the demands of normal daily activity. An individual who is fit, or committed to regular exercise, displays characteristics that differ from those who are unfit. Broadly, these changes evolve from an ability to exercise at a higher level, and also to recover from hard physical activity faster than those who are unfit do. To raise one's level of fitness requires a commitment of both time and effort. And it demands an acceptance that during the early stages at least one must endure a certain measure of physical discomfort. In a determination to clear these early hurdles, there needs to be an appreciation of the benefits that accrue from being fit and how these can best be achieved. These statements are just as relevant in retirement as they were when we were younger. Fitness is not going to be a miracle cure for all the physiological difficulties which accompany old age but it will certainly prolong an active life and stave off dependence for several years.

Exercise in old age

Exercise capacity declines by approximately 10% for each decade after 30 years of age. However, the extent to which this reflects a disinclination to take exercise with advancing years, is not clear. Ageing is naturally associated with loss of muscle mass, by the age of 80 approximately 50% of normal adult muscle mass has been lost. This is reflected as a loss of strength. However, there is no doubt that both fitness levels and strength increase with regular exercise and, what is more, they show the greatest improvements in people who have been exercising least. They also show the greatest decline in those who are very active, but who are forced to rest, through injury or illness for example. This was beautifully demonstrated by the distinguished Swedish physiologist, Bengt Saltin, who took five male volunteers aged 19–21 and subjected them to a 20-day period of bed rest followed by 50 days of training. As an indication of fitness, oxygen consumption fell by an average of 20% following the period of rest, and took over two months to return to pre-rest levels. This has a sobering effect when you consider how often old-age illnesses require bed-rest. The good news is that, even in very old people, fitness can be improved by gentle regular exercise – it can mean the difference between being able to get out of bed in the morning, doing your own shopping, cleaning and cooking, and needing a carer to help with these simple everyday tasks.

The ability to exercise is determined largely by state of health and much less so by age. Thus, when making decisions about prescribing exercise, two factors must be borne in mind. First, what is the level of activity to which the you are accustomed and second, bearing in mind the state of health, what level of exercise can be achieved. In its position statement the American College of Sports Medicine recommends "At least 20–30 minutes of continuous or intermittent aerobic activity should be taken 3–5 days per week", a target easily surpassed by some though beyond the reach of many others.

The important thing about taking exercise is that it should become a habit. And to do that it needs to be enjoyable, and taken in the company of others. The exercise prescription must also take account of people with special needs, such as those with chronic bronchitis, arterial disease, obesity or diabetes. It also needs to be tailored to those who are recovering from injury or illness.

Misconceptions about exercise

A recent letter in the *British Medical Journal* reveals a worrying trend in older people's attitudes to exercise and the consequences upon their health:

> Four out of 10 people older than 50 are totally inactive, yet over half of sedentary people in this age group believe that they take part in enough physical activity to keep fit … For the frailest older people, being sedentary is a greater risk than being active, but carers and professionals may encourage individual people to be less active.
>
> P Simey, D Skelton. *BMJ* 2001; **322**: 796.

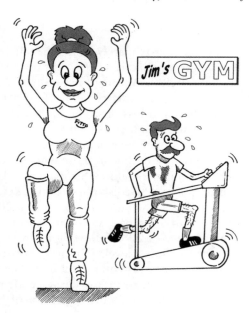

The letter was in response to a previous article, *A healthy old age: realistic or futile goal?* by Professor Marion Mundo (*BMJ* 2000; **321**: 1149–1151). She observes that older people do not imagine that they can achieve the stereotypical image of proper "exercise" such as a long run, a sweaty session in a gym or a fast furious game of squash, so they don't bother. It is time for society's attitudes towards old age to change substantially and to encourage activity rather than perpetuating the concept of retirement being the time to "put your feet up"; for example, Mundo warns that, "Well-intentioned relatives who take over the household chores may be depriving their elderly relative of their main activity of the week".

Obesity, exercise and diet

Obesity is a major problem in advancing years. Grossly obese people cannot exercise because they cannot carry the weight. What is more, they cannot lose the heat. And those who don't exercise cannot lose weight: a case of double jeopardy! Body mass index (BMI kg/m^2), is used to estimate excess weight in adults. "Overweight" is defined as a BMI greater than 25. The World Health Organisation have compiled a risk index of co-morbidity by country, classifying those with a BMI over 30 as high risk, and over 40 as very high risk. The British are now the fattest people in Europe, just ahead of the Germans, with 17% of male and 20% of female adults having a BMI in excess of thirty. Twenty years ago, only around 7% of Britains were obese.

Obese people don't necessarily eat a lot, but they do eat more than they need. Research has also shown that the obese move about less than those who are lean. Calorie restriction without a concomitant increase in physical activity is seldom successful in achieving substantial weight loss, but nonetheless dietary considerations are important. During their arduous training course it has been estimated that the average Royal Marine will require a daily intake of more than 7,000 calories simply to maintain body weight; in comparison, some sedentary individuals may gain weight with a daily intake of less than 1,500 calories.

Ideally up to 60% of the calories consumed should be in the form of complex carbohydrate such as potato or pasta, with less than 30% fat. The greater part should be eaten at breakfast time or in the early part of the day, with only a carbohydrate snack taken before retiring. Calorie for calorie, carbohydrate occupies about four times the volume of fat, so a diet rich in carbohydrate is more likely to satisfy appetite, because it provides greater bulk.

What are the health benefits of regular exercise?

In March 2002, the *New England Journal of Medicine* carried an article which provided evidence regarding the relationship between fitness and survival of cardiovascular disease. The study enrolled over 6,000 male subjects referred for clinical exercise testing, 3,600 of whom had coronary artery disease, heart failure, peripheral vascular disease or an abnormal exercise ECG and were categorised as having cardiovascular disease. The participants' exercise capacity was measured in metabolic equivalents (MET; 1 MET=the rate of oxygen consumption at rest, i.e. 3–4 ml per kilo per minute). After a mean follow-up period of six months, 1256 subjects had died from various causes but the observations from analysing which participants had died were astonishing: as fitness levels increased, a near linear reduction in mortality was observed. Each single MET increase in exercise capacity conferred a 12% improvement in survival. The risk of death amongst those with a low peak exercise capacity (<5 MET) was nearly double that of fitter participants with higher peak exercise capacities (>8 MET). And the relative risk for the least fit people was four times higher than that of the fittest subjects, whether or not they had cardiovascular disease. So, the case in favour of getting fit could not be more compelling.

There is now evidence that for those with hypertension, regular exercise can reduce diastolic blood pressure by an average of 7 mmHg. Exercise is also an effective way of controlling obesity, if linked with appropriate calorie restriction. More is also emerging about a reduction in the incidence of myocardial infarction and stroke. Other benefits of exercise include reduced risk of diabetes and cancers, a reduction in the rate of osteoporosis-linked bone loss, reduced joint and muscle pain, and exercise helps to maintain better balance skills which reduce the risk of injuries through falls. Regular exercise is associated with greater mental well-being too, it can provide relief during depressive episodes, and better control over one's motor skills naturally improves confidence. In addition, the mere fact of prolonging independence from medical and social care must be a huge incentive to all of us as we face old age. Walking, gardening and golf, as examples, bring with them opportunities to socialise, to enjoy the countryside and breathe lungfuls of fresh air. What better prescription could you recommend yourself?

Further information

- *Physical activity for patients; an exercise prescription* – Royal College of Physicians, London (ISBN 1-86016-128-6); website: www.rcplondon.ac.uk
- *Exercise for Healthy Ageing: exercise programmes proven in research to increase muscle strength* – Dr Dawn Skelton (ISBN 0-95253-261-1) for Research in Ageing, PO Box 32833, London N1 9ZQ; telephone: 020 7843 1550; website: www.ageing.org/publications
- *Better health in retirement* – Dr Anne Roberts (ISBN 0-86242-251-5) for Age Concern, Age Concern Books, PO Box 232, Newton Abbot, Devon, TQ12 4XQ; telephone: 0870 44 22 044; website: www.ageconcern.org.uk
- ActivAge UK organises over 100 projects nationwide to encourage activity and fitness for older people. Contact: ActivAge Unit, Age Concern England, Astral House, 1268 London Road, London SW16 4ER; telephone: 020 8765 7231; website: www.activage.org.uk
- Myers J, Prakash M, Froelicher V, Do D *et al*. Exercise capacity and mortality among men referred for exercise testing *N Engl J Med* 2002; **346**: 793–801.

CHAPTER 6

Lifestyle

To get back to my youth I would do anything in the world, except get up early or be respectable

Oscar Wilde (1854–1900) *The Picture of Dorian Gray*

The word "lifestyle" does not appear in the fourth edition of the *Concise Oxford Dictionary* published in 1950. Later editions define this word as "an individual's way of life". The youth of the word is easily explained as it was only in the last half century that we saw general acceptance that much morbidity and mortality is self-induced and serious efforts made to evaluate the risks that caused it. Of course there had been faltering steps earlier and Sir William Osler (1849–1919) stressed the importance of rest, food, fresh air and exercise but it was only in 1963 that the full implications of cigarette-smoking were appreciated; until then the pea-soup fogs so vividly described by Charles Dickens had obscured its importance. In the early 1950s a performance at Sadler's Wells was cancelled because smog made the stage invisible from the dress circle. Smokeless fuel made for cleaner air but still diseases of the respiratory and cardiovascular systems obstinately ravaged those who smoked cigarettes.

In retirement the golden rules for a healthy lifestyle do not change, but as we age they must be observed stringently. Much of the disease of younger people and those in middle-age seems in the present state of our knowledge to be due to either faulty genes or bad luck; to remain well over 60 is often the result of good management and close attention to those golden rules. In a busy working life, short cuts will have been taken: hurriedly eaten meals of poor quality in hospital canteens are bad for digestion and disturbed sleep patterns leave little time for exercise or for hobbies. Which doctor, hurrying in the morning to hospital or surgery, has not ignored the gastro-colic reflex? In retirement, there will be time to answer its call just as there will be time to attend a Weight Watchers' class, time to visit a farmers' market to buy healthy organic food, time to take long country walks or to swim, time even to brush the teeth thoroughly – time, in short, to lead a healthy life after the long years of medical practice, which by its nature sits uneasily with routine and is so disruptive of habit.

At the point of retirement the doctor may have as much as one-third of his adult life still to come. During the last century the expectation of life increased by almost twenty-five years. With this prospect ahead it is essential to adopt a positive attitude of "the best is yet to come" rather than "the party's over now".

This is the moment for an audit of our own health which doctors so often neglect. Am I overweight? Do I eat a healthy diet? Am I hypertensive? Can I walk three miles in one hour without difficulty? If not, why not? Do I do so regularly? Do I sleep well? Do I drink too much alcohol? Do I smoke cigarettes? Am I contented? Is my spouse or partner contented? Do we live happily together?

Each of us knows an individual who defies all the rules, who has the figure of Falstaff, who has never refused a drink or cigar, who takes no exercise and eats pudding drenched in cream and Cointreau, who lives to 90 and is killed in a road traffic accident. But the Life Assurers of Edinburgh and Glasgow know that this is luck and the statistics gleaned by epidemiologists all over the world prove it. Since the late 1970s the insurance companies have offered rates to non-smokers which are the same as those for smokers four years younger. They are more inclined now to load the premium for obesity, for moderately raised blood pressure, impaired carbohydrate metabolism, excess alcohol consumption and a past history of psychiatric disturbance. The canny Scottish underwriters know a risk when they see one.

The risk factors interact with each other and often two or more play their part in pathogenesis. Smoking, obesity, a diet rich in saturated fats, hypertension and diabetes all have a role in arterial disease; one third of deaths are due to coronary artery disease and a further one sixth are due to cerebro-vascular accident.

Smoking

Most authorities regard smoking as the risk factor which results in more years lost than any other. Its effects are too well-known to itemise here but an astonishing number of sensible and intelligent patients still claim, when in advanced stages of cardiovascular or respiratory disease, that no physician has asked them whether they smoke cigarettes. Possibly this is because physicians who themselves smoke are in denial. There is help available: psychotherapy, self-help groups, nicotine chewing gum and patches – but there is no substitute for willpower. Smoking is expensive: twenty cigarettes a day costs between £1,000 and £1,500 per year. Much of the excess mortality of smoking, particularly that due to cardiovascular disorders, is removed quite soon after quitting the habit.

Obesity

Obesity is commoner now than in the past. A century ago men died of want; today they die of plenty and much packaged food (which is high in sugar, salt and fat, low in fibre) should be regarded as a dangerous pathogen. It is instructive to inspect the shopping baskets at the supermarket check-out, their contents often correlate closely with the figures carrying them. Obesity plays its part in many diseases including hypertension, arterial disorders, diabetes, gout, osteoarthritis, hiatus hernia, hyperlipidaemia and gallstones. It renders the subject less suitable for surgery, more prone to accidents and presents formidable nursing problems in serious or terminal illness. As the body mass index (BMI) is difficult to calculate, it is simpler to measure girth: waist circumference should be less than 102 cm in a man and 88 cm in a woman. This recognises the particular risks attached to intra-abdominal fat. Weight loss should be accomplished by limiting intake of food and increasing exercise. In the animal kingdom only man and domestic animals become obese, others eat when hungry. An old English aphorism instructs us to "breakfast like a king, lunch like a prince and dine like a pauper" – it seems sensible to eat more before periods of maximum exertion. The aim should be to lose weight slowly, say 1–2 lb per week.

Exercise

Exercise can be in any form and should be enjoyable, but it should be sufficiently vigorous to cause slight dyspnoea and sweating and to raise the pulse rate. Twice a week it should be prolonged to take advantage of the aerobic metabolism that begins after about 20 minutes. Walking is particularly advantageous for those with osteoporosis; swimming for those with early osteoarthritis of the weight-bearing joints. If walking is the main activity it should be sufficiently brisk to cause mild breathlessness on hills or if talking to a friend. A daily walk of half an hour with a longer one twice a week is a good target. Golf has been called "a

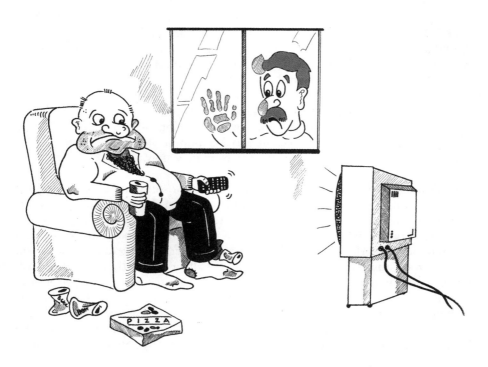

good walk spoilt" and if a dog is your companion it should be trained not to stop at every lamp-post, nor chase every rabbit in the county. It is advisable to have several forms of exercise to encourage suppleness, stamina and strength.

Diet

Diet has been too much ignored in the past by English doctors – to the French *"La Régime"* has always been an important part of overall care and we have been slow to follow. In the present state of knowledge the ideal diet should supply sufficient calories to maintain the correct body weight for height and age, and it should be low in saturated fats and high in fibre. Red meat, dairy produce and eggs should be limited and poultry and fish eaten more often. Oily fish containing omega oils which are anti-oxidants also supply essential amino acids: sardines, pilchards, anchovies, salmon, trout and mackerel provide plenty of variety. White fish like cod, halibut, turbot, sole and plaice provide protein but beware the chips that partner them. The hidden fat in cakes and pastries should be avoided. Lipid levels should be measured and it is likely that most doctors will have done this before retirement, if only out of curiosity. A full lasting lipid profile should be ordered with breakdown of high density lipids, low density lipids and triglycerides. A few people will have congenital hyperlipidaemia, but lesser degrees should be corrected by low fat diet, weight loss where appropriate and extra exercise but some stubborn cases will need treatment with statins.

Dietary fibre protects the alimentary tract from many disorders as well as having wider significance. Although Cleave and later Burkitt are widely credited with revealing the benefit of fibre, its importance was observed by Dean Swift (1667–1745) two centuries earlier in his book *Ordure*, a slim volume less widely read than his *Gulliver's Travels*. Byron, too, knew the importance of keeping his bowels open, for in the downstairs lavatory at Newstead Abbey, the visitor may read his Lordship's thoughts on the subject:

> O Cloacina, Goddess of this place,
> Look on thy subject with a smiling face
> Soft and obedient may his motions flow
> Not rashly swift nor obstinately slow.

The ideal diet should include enough fibre to give a soft and bulky but formed stool, the consistency of toothpaste and one that floats in the lavatory pan, for fibre gives buoyancy. Useful sources of fibre are pulses, beans, peas, broccoli, cabbage, root vegetables and most fruit. Wholemeal bread contains nine times the fibre of white *Mother's Pride*. A visit to a farmers' market on a Sunday will provide good hunting for fibre seekers and, equally importantly, supports British farming. Salt must be restricted only in those with a tendency to hypertension. *Lo-Salt* is palatable and supplies potassium in place of sodium. Tinned foods contain much salt used as a preservative.

Alcohol is beneficial providing the guidelines are observed, but should be limited if the subject is either obese or hypertensive. Red wine contains anti-oxidants and is the most nutritious form in which it can be taken. Shakespeare refers to the "merry cheerer of the heart" and Keats, in his days as an apothecary's apprentice, wrote to his brother and sister extolling the virtues of claret, "You do not feel it quarrelling with one's liver. No, 'tis rather a peacemaker and lies as quiet as it did in the grape". There must, of course, be no question of taking alcohol before driving or using machinery such as a chain-saw. As little as one unit of alcohol can impair judgement.

Sleep

Sleep may have been disturbed often in a life of medical practice. A real effort should be made to get off the sleeping pills to which many doctors are addicted. No longer does it matter if they don't sleep for a night or two. How much better a night cap and how much more enjoyable! Sleep should improve with regular exercise and with less anxiety over professional matters. An optimistic approach to life is naturally a great bonus in retirement. Though it is unlikely that our personality will change greatly after the age of 60, many recently retired doctors are surprised at the new lease of life stimulated by increased travel, old hobbies revisited, interests rediscovered and more time for friendship and social activities. It seems particularly beneficial to have one physical hobby like gardening or long-distance walking and a cerebral one involving study and research – they complement each other. For example, holidays can be arranged with companies like Alternative Travel or Inn-Travel, who move the walkers' luggage from inn to inn; these can be tailored to the individual capabilities of distance, energy and enthusiasm.

There will be joy and contentment in spending more time with a partner or spouse if both remain well and fit, but that is to encroach on the territory of other contributors. Above all life must be fun. We all know from simple observation of our patients that it is often the *joie de vivre* which acts like a dynamo on the human body and is more important than eating raw carrots, jogging in the rain or refusing puddings. Life must remain exciting and novel, for it is the *new* experiences that keep us young at heart. Dame Sybil Thorndike, aged 80, danced and sang in a musical version of *Vanity Fair* in November 1962. The show flopped but she gamely told the press, "One should never be sorry one has attempted something new – never, never, never!" She died, aged 94, fourteen years later – that must be a lesson for all of us.

DH

CHAPTER 7

Continuing part-time work

Putting it in context

Historically, retirement was something which happened at the age of sixty-five, whatever your occupation. To some, it was a blessed release from a life of unfulfilled drudgery, while to others it was the curtain coming down on a life they loved, with the horrifying prospect of miserable boredom until they died! Both are rather extreme scenarios, but were not all that unknown.

Today, the situation is very different. Apart from anything else, there is a much more relaxed attitude to the timing of retirement. Twenty to thirty years ago, taking retirement *before* the age of sixty-five, apart from as a result of ill-health, was viewed with suspicion. "Why is he giving up?", "Is he deserting the Health Service?", "Can he no longer cope?", "Is he just out to make more money elsewhere?". It is now accepted that there is nothing magical or sacrosanct about deferring retirement to the age of sixty-five or in changing a career pathway at any time. Doctors no longer feel morally obliged or compelled to continue in a post until a rigid statutory retirement age. Indeed, more and more are electing to retire from the NHS in their late fifties or early sixties. A consequence of this is that many are still very full of vim and vigour and keen to continue in some form of work.

The purpose of this book is to examine all sorts of aspects of retirement from medicine. I have chosen to interpret this as retirement from the NHS and, in particular, retirement of the hospital consultant. I am not qualified to comment on "what it takes" for retirement from general practice or administrative appointments – a wholly different ball game. This chapter considers the implications and practicality of continuing part-time work in some area of medical practice after retirement from an NHS appointment.

What are the options?

Continuing to do some form of part-time medical practice after retirement from the NHS boils down to four or five main areas of activity:

- clinical practice in the private sector
- medico-legal work
- sitting on tribunals or appeals committees
- working abroad

- voluntary work as, for example, with St John's Ambulance or as a medical advisor to an aid agency.

With the possible exception of working abroad, these are not mutually exclusive.

How do you choose?

In general, the area of medical practice pursued after retirement is conditioned by the nature of the NHS appointment prior to retirement and whether or not non-NHS work had been carried out. It is also conditioned by forward planning. Thus, it is relatively easy for the consultant who has been engaged in private practice alongside NHS work to simply give up an NHS appointment and continue with private practice on a part-time basis. It is much more difficult for the full-time NHS consultant or academic, who has done little or no private practice, suddenly to attempt to establish a part-time private practice on retiring from an NHS or university appointment. It is wise for the latter to plan ahead as to what they might do on retirement.

That said, the situation is altering rapidly. Twenty years ago, academics were not allowed, or were actively discouraged from, involvement in private practice. This has changed dramatically and indeed many teaching hospitals seem to encourage private practice by their academic staff as an extra source of earnings and provide facilities for this. Academics thus have much more experience of the workings of the private sector.

A medico-legal practice is also not something which can suddenly be embarked upon when retiring from the NHS but something that is built up over many years. It has the advantage of not requiring much in the way of office or clinic facilities, although it will be usual to have at least one consultation with the client.

Sitting on tribunals or various appeals committees does appear to be something which can be taken up *de nova* on retirement, but selection to sit on these seems to depend on some old boy network. It is not so much you electing to do it, but rather being offered a job! Often involving travel around the country, this area of medical specialisation is not unattractive.

Medical work overseas after retirement from the NHS seems to fall in to two areas. There are those who have had previous experience of doing medical work in developing countries, some, but not all, in medical missionary environments. Of these, some feel strongly that they would like to make a final contribution before they give up medical practice completely. At the invitation of former colleagues, they return to hospitals or countries where they have worked previously to do teaching and to give part-time clinical assistance, as well as helping to update medical practice. Depending on the country, it is generally not financially rewarding. Talking to those who have done this, all too often the story is one of great sadness at the progressive decline in health care facilities in deprived countries.

The other group who go abroad on retirement are the academics. There is considerable attraction in giving up your professorship early to go abroad to a medical school where you can make a significant contribution to medical education and practice without the departmental hassles of British university life. Commonly, the financial inducements are not unattractive. For many academics with no interest in private practice but a real passion for teaching, this is a very attractive finale to a long commitment to medical education. It does, however, make huge demands on their personal life. How many, even the most devoted, partners are prepared to uproot their familiar, comfortable home at the age of sixty-plus to go and live in a foreign land where, all too often, women have a different cultural status? This option is much easier for the single medic with no close family commitments.

Voluntary work can be very rewarding. It is very much determined by the motivation and enthusiasm of the individual. It may be a continuation of voluntary work carried out in parallel with an NHS appointment, or something taken up in retirement.

Do you have what is needed?

As mentioned already, electing to continue in part-time work after retiring from the NHS is not all that simple. Choices are heavily weighted by previous experience and forward planning over some time. This is especially important in undertaking private practice after retirement. For this reason, it is worth looking in more detail at the various factors which can condition the potential for doing such work.

The requirements for private practice

There are certain basic requirements for running a viable and rewarding private practice. You must have a consulting room. Traditionally, those embarking on private practice at an early stage in their careers either rented consulting rooms in a part of town recognised as the hub of private practice, set up private consultation in their own homes, or hired private consulting rooms in a hospital or clinic. These latter might be NHS or private hospitals.

Those already engaged in private practice at retirement will have consulting rooms in which they can continue. A possible exception are those who have used consulting rooms in an NHS hospital which are no longer available. For these latter consultants and those electing to start private practice after retirement, the major factor in obtaining consulting rooms is cost. Renting rooms or converting space in your own home is not cheap. It demands a reasonable number of patients to make it financially viable. A safer alternative is to use the out-patient consulting facilities now offered by many private hospitals. These may be used *ad hoc* or on a regular sessional basis depending on the activity of the practice.

In the past, there was some resistance to having consulting rooms in a private hospital, as it was suggested that this tied the consultant to having all investigations done by that hospital as well as using its hospital beds. Some patients felt there was more freedom for the consultant working from his own rooms and, in turn, more choice for them despite the obvious advantage of having both the consultation and the investigations done under the same roof. The use of consulting rooms in private hospitals has now become so widespread that these concerns have waned, especially as consultants do not feel constrained to have investigations done "in house" if they feel this inappropriate. Nor do they feel obliged to admit patients exclusively to the hospital. Use of these facilities seems the most rational approach for those without established consulting rooms.

The second essential for private practice is that you have a regular supply of patients! Private practices are most often built up over several years. To those already doing private practice on retirement, this should not be a problem. For those who have done little or no private work before retirement, it can be a major limiting factor as there is a minimal referral rate below which the practice is not financially viable.

Acquiring an active practice is not easy. Some "inherit" practices from older retiring colleagues but this usually happens to younger consultants with the reasonable expectation of many years of practice to come. Referral is very dependent on colleagues and especially general practitioners. In London and other major cities, there is also referral from the medical attachés of various foreign embassies. The key to getting referrals is "spreading the word" as widely as possible. Direct advertising is not yet acceptable, but "change of address" cards are in common use. Many private hospitals also now publish details of consultants seeing patients on their premises. It is, nevertheless, often a slow process acquiring patients!

Private practice also requires admitting facilities to private hospitals. Application must be made for these and these applications will be vetted by the Medical Staff Committee. It is unusual to have admitting facilities denied unless it is felt there are already too many consultants with admitting rights in a particular field.

So far, the orientation is toward clinical practice. Consultants in specialist fields, such as radiology, pathology, bacteriology, also do private work. In general, they seem to enter the private practice field quite early in their careers in the NHS and regularly continue after retirement from the NHS. A few in shortage specialties take up private work late in their careers, when they simply move into vacant slots.

Secretarial assistance is essential – medical practice, whether clinical or medico-legal, can generate a great deal of typing! In addition, running a successful private practice requires that there is easy access for referring doctors or patients to some central co-ordinator. This is why the good practice secretary is worth their weight in gold. If doing part-time clinical work, careful thought must be given to who this would be and who will deal with the reports and correspondence. All too often, these last two roles are dumped on the wife or partner. Failure for GPs or patients to have easy access to a consultant means the practice will fade away.

Ease of access to the consultant, especially when setting out in private practice, is also important when requests are made for him or her to advise on in-patients. If well organised, the retired part-time clinician can score here as, without NHS clinics or ward rounds, they can commonly arrange to see an in-patient quickly. It is all about availability and ease of contact.

Financial considerations

Clearly, whenever retirement is taken, it is essential to consider the financial implications, "Do I have enough to live on or must I go on earning money?" This must be a very personal assessment dependent on all sorts of social and domestic factors. NHS retirement pensions, especially if boosted by merit awards, are pretty generous. Many consultants, with lots of years of service, can afford to retire early and not be financially disadvantaged. It is, however, wise to check with the BMA exactly what your pension should be if considering retiring and to what extent waiting another few years might significantly increase the pension. Hanging around in your sixties for an increased merit award can be pretty dodgy!

I suspect that most clinicians taking early retirement do not really need a boost to their pensions. Any extra earnings is cream on the top. Most go on in private practice because they love it!

Have you got what it takes?

For most of my professional career, I held a full-time appointment, initially fully university and later combined university and NHS. In my early fifties I decided that I did not wish to continue with what was, in effect, a full-time career, and, in particular, I did not wish to become increasingly engaged with university and other outside committees which was the usual way forward. I dreaded giving up active involvement in day-to-day patient care. For this reason, I elected to drop to a maximal part-time NHS appointment and embark on private practice.

Pre-retirement, I never had, nor did I strive for, a big private practice. In considerable measure this was because I never really resolved the competing demands of my busy NHS post and the demands of private practice. The former tend to win outright. Taking early retirement from the NHS and a big successful department at the age of sixty-one was a shock, but in terms of part-time private practice a great liberation. I had well-established, shared rooms in Harley Street, an excellent part-time secretary and a congenial, if not enormous, practice. Consulting three half days a week kept me and the practice happy. Because of one's new found freedom, one could also see emergency patients at other times. Requests to see patients in various hospitals became easy and indeed positively pleasurable. I was never under-occupied and never bored. I had always done a little medico-legal work and this continued and indeed increased.

Probably the most profound effect on me as a result of retiring from the NHS and continuing in private practice was that I no longer felt guilty! Previously, I had always felt bad if I deserted some NHS session to rush off to see an ill patient in the private sector or vice versa. Now there was no challenge of loyalties. It also allowed me really to commit my energies to one sector of medical practice.

The down side of retiring from a busy, pretty high-powered teaching hospital post to continue medical practice in the private sector, was the sense of isolation. Throughout my professional career I had been part of a medical team and engaged in research. There was always input from all members of the team in making diagnoses, deciding on best treatment and predicting outcome. Regular sessions with research fellows and regular departmental and hospital meetings stimulated and educated the mind. There is no doubt that consultants are kept on their toes by bright young members of the team and kept up to date.

Consultants must keep ahead of the game if they are to retain credibility. On your own in private practice you risk losing this and have to work deliberately hard to keep up to date – read the journals, go to speciality meetings, and keep attending clinical presentations. Even doing this, it is never the same as the stimulation and, indeed, education from ward rounds and research meetings. I found this hard to cope with if I was to convince myself that I really was at the front of medical practice. Failure to keep up is probably the main indicator that it is time to stop clinical practice.

WRC

CHAPTER 8

Continuing professional associations and life-long learning

R etirement is a new career. Not so arduous perhaps as the one you are leaving nor so destructive of your social life but still a career in which you must be positively engaged, it must be planned and learning will be part of it. The golf course and the river bank, the boat and the beach all have their attractions but they will not be enough. You are probably looking forward to 20 years of active life and you must use your mind or lose it. Life-long learning should not be just a pious hope, it should simply be short-hand for a practical programme which is remarkably good for your intellectual health. Perhaps you feel that, after 40 years of keeping up with the rapidly advancing medical field, you need a rest from studying. You would be wrong – what you need is a redirection of your study.

Perhaps you are fortunate enough to possess talents in art or music and have now the opportunity to develop your skills but even that is a process which itself requires a structured learning programme. You must not be content with repetition of your old masterpieces. If you have those practical skills so popular with the family such as DIY or furniture restoration by all means exercise them but you must still learn to extend your scope. These are hobbies but for all of us, dexterous or ham-handed, there is surprising satisfaction to be gained from new adventures in the academic field, from re-engaging the education mode and gaining an understanding of a subject beyond our previous expertise.

You have, of course, time to look around and find the subject which attracts you and the milieu in which you can best pursue your study, but procrastination is dangerous and aimless drifting can too easily take over. You may choose to utilise your present background and contacts as a starting point for the academic exploration of some fascinating byways within the larger medical field. On the other hand you may feel that a sharp break from the past is essential and that further involvement in medicine is abhorrent, in which case the opportunities are bewilderingly numerous. Start looking!

Continuing professional connections

At the point of retirement you will find yourself a member of numerous medical societies, medico-political or specialist associations, study groups, dining or travelling clubs and you probably retain some connection with a Royal College. You have to consider what part these will play in your new career. You may well look askance at their exorbitant subscription rates but they will probably offer you senior or, if you are lucky, honorary membership. That still leaves the cost of conferences which will seem outrageous once they cannot be claimed against income tax. Do not resign in a hurry – these contacts will be vital if you plan anything with a medical connection, but even if you are making a clean break with the past, a society provides you with a circle of friends with whom it would be too easy to lose contact. Remember,

> Senescence begins,
> And middle age ends,
> On the day your descendents
> Outnumber your friends.

Your role in the societies will inevitably change with your retirement and that is something to which you must adapt. You may have worked hard and have had a pivotal role as councillor, secretary or finally as president but others are now filling these posts – they will probably change all the policies and procedures that you had pioneered, which is vexing, but put a brave face on it! Better to be the elder statesman consulted with deference if not with agreement than to become "*difficilis, querulus laudator temporis acti*". Congratulate your successors if they succeed, enjoy a private smile if they fail. There are still useful and important jobs to do in these colleges or societies, in the library, the archives or the museum. You can organize social events and outings for the elderly! You can write the history of the society or at least the obituaries of your friends.

You may value the societies as a way of following from the side lines the development of your own specialty but be cautious about expressing your opinions. Your knowledge is no doubt at its pinnacle and there is some aspect upon which you are the acknowledged authority but remember that pre-eminence wastes with horrifying rapidity. If you have an eponymous lecture to give or a book to write, do it now! It was an object lesson when I was once bequeathed a case of unsold copies of a book by a man whose experience was unrivalled and whose capacity for assimilating information seemed remarkable but who devoted five years to working up his material, and took a further two to get it through the publishers. It dropped, as they say, still-born from the press.

The medico-political field is at least as subject to change as the academic. The inflow of information ceases abruptly when you leave office and it is dangerous to assume that your views will be valued once you lack a mastery of contemporary detail. But if your new learning programme is related to the medical field, history, ethics or comparative medicine for instance, the facilities of the college and the societies are invaluable and you will have something positive to contribute to their meetings.

The business of learning

So you are embarking on a course of life-long learning! In the 20 years you are looking forward to there will be time for many things but you must begin by choosing a subject which will suit your lifestyle. It should be a voyage of discovery which will get you physically and intellectually away from your usual haunts. It should bring you into contact with others who share your interest but who are preferably from a different age group and background. It should require an active as well as a passive learning process, you must produce something, publish something, pass an exam or publicly air your expertise. Perhaps in the second decade of your retirement you can afford to be a little more relaxed but in the first you must work at it. Even with these provisos the possibilities seem endless but here are a few ideas.

Learning a foreign language and studying its literature presents an attractive option offering encouragement to travel while you are still fit as well as ample reading matter when the time comes to put your feet up. The history of art is popular, almost too popular with those who lack the skill to practise it, for there is a danger in allowing viewing of galleries and listening to lectures to become the easy alternative to active study. The history of medicine or science is increasingly chosen by a diversity of students from outside the profession but the history of almost anything has its fascination.

Genealogy can be intriguing and facilities for it are increasingly available. You will have to follow up very many lines in your family if the study is going to last you a life time, but even if you find that your ancestors were a depressingly undistinguished lot you can at least reflect that it is better to have come up in the world than to have gone down.

Archaeology takes you into the prehistory and can have a practical element if you don't mind digging. Architecture presents you with something to admire or detest but importantly it demands that you travel around to look at it. Geology offers opportunities for exploration but for this, as for other sciences, you may need to brush up on your basics first – quantum physics has moved on a bit since you took your A-levels. Botany sounds rather old-fashioned but goes well with your gardening. Photography can be involved in almost any subject but can be a study in itself. If you are already a collector you may well want to take on the detailed study of antiques, ceramics, books or clocks or whatever it is you collect and there is plenty of scope for learning as well as rummaging in junk shops and auction rooms. For the truly dedicated academics there are the abstruse pleasures of philosophy and ethics or the intricacies of higher mathematics.

Whatever your choice, you will have to start with a formal course of instruction. It is theoretically possible to read yourself into your subject in the privacy of your study but in practice the pressures of family and social life and the call of the great outdoors will prevent you from getting to grips with it. Theoretically there are book-lined studies with a computer but no television, where the reader is immune to urgent demands to mow the lawn or mend a fuse; there are texts so riveting that the attraction cannot wander nor the eyelids droop; there are those even in the seventh decade of life who after a day in the fresh air can settle down to work with the same determination of a student reading for his fellowship. In practice it must be admitted that it will be only by subjecting yourself to the discipline of an educational course that you will be able to prepare yourself for the lasting enjoyment of your special interest.

Courses may last three years or three months, they may be arduous or easy but they are indispensable for the serious business of your new career. Once you are through with them you will derive lasting pleasure from your new expertise. You will be a member of the relevant societies, you will receive the relevant journals, go on the relevant trips, and start your own explorations or research.

Where to study?

Where will you go for your course? For medically related subjects there will be no difficulty. The societies and medical schools you already know can provide what you need. The Worshipful Society of Apothecaries runs an admirable *History of Medicine* diploma course in association with the Wellcome Trust. You can then enrol with the "Friends of the Wellcome Library and Centre" and attend the lectures and seminars which the Wellcome Centre itself puts on throughout the academic year. For non-medical courses the local public library can give you all the relevant addresses; it will load you with leaflets and advertising material for courses on everything practical and some things academic.

Local adult education colleges are mostly concerned with the practical skills required by young adults furthering their careers and classes are often in the evenings. If you need to sharpen your technique in your workshop, garage or garden these may suit you but for a start on a programme of life-long learning you must go elsewhere. A good place to start searching is through the *Hot Courses* publication, available in most newsagents and on the web at www.hotcourses.com. This contains details for over 465,000 courses across the UK. In London, the City Lit Institute offers lecture courses on many subjects but they are mostly for passive learning. You might take one as a taster before delving deeper into your interest. If you are thinking of writing your memoirs, for example, it might be as well to attend one of their many courses on aspects of creative writing.

Universities and learned societies are the obvious places for academic study and many like Birkbeck College in the University of London now offer part-time courses in a variety of subjects at a standard appropriate for you. Your medical degrees will ordinarily exempt you from other entry requirements but for advanced subjects unrelated to medicine you may need to take a foundation course. Universities aim to award degrees or diplomas and although you may not now need any more letters after your name why not aim to complete these courses. Attending regular lectures and tutorials for three academic years may seem fairly daunting but it will obviously be correspondingly rewarding. A friend of mine took a full course in German literature and found that the most trying part of it was travelling into Oxford from his delightful farmhouse in the Cotswolds! Working alongside students much less than half his age was as enjoyable and as enlightening as grappling with the complexity of syntax and the tortuous imagery of German authors.

For most retirees the Open University offers a more accessible but in no sense an inferior educational experience. The fees and the entry qualifications are modest and most of the work can be done at home. Regular tutorials keep you in touch with the lecturers and a week or two at a summer school gives you a view of your fellow students. The printed course material supplied is of high quality, in fact it is now often used surreptitiously by those at more prestigious institutions. Some programmes are transmitted by the BBC in the early morning and others are taught by the video tapes they send you. Regular written work is required from you and inevitably there is an exam at the end of the year. A degree can be obtained by a series of modules taken over three years or you can pick and choose among a wide diversity of subjects on offer. Computer literacy is essential for most of the science courses but this should not be a problem for the coming generation of retirees; if there are any unreconstructed pen and paper dinosaurs they will have to start by learning the keyboard, the screen and the mouse.

What about the exam? There are doctors who claim to have been so badly traumatized by their experiences in youth that any prospect of an exam is a complete turn off. It is true that you can enjoy the course (and forgo the letters after your name), without attempting the final hurdle but most feel that they must accept the challenge and find that the sense of satisfaction in passing more than compensates for the effort involved.

The University of the Third Age (U3A) may suit those who like to be more relaxed about their learning or who have passed through the degree course but want to keep in touch. U3A is tailored for the retired, with branches in many areas. It organises lectures and meetings, usually in the day time, for small groups and often in private homes. It costs very little, requires no entry qualifications, sets no exams and awards no diplomas but can provide a satisfying educational experience. It caters for the special interests of members who want to teach as well as learn. An acquaintance of mine was a retired professor of radiation physics who thoroughly enjoyed lecturing on the metaphysical theories of the modern philosophers he had studied with the U3A.

The course, long or short, whether for a degree, a diploma or something much less formidable, is the beginning of your learning programme. Just as your medical education provided the basis for the understanding of a fascinating and rapidly changing subject, some aspect of which has intrigued you for 40 years, your new expertise will mature over the next 20 without the stress but with all the interest of your first career. So bite the bullet and enrol in a course. Good luck!

DIW

Further information

- The History of Medicine diploma course – website:
  www.apothecaries.org.uk or telephone: 0207 236 1180 for details

- The CityLit Institute website: www.citylit.ac.uk or telephone 0207 7430 0543 for advice and information
- Birkbeck College in the University of London website: www.bbk.ac.uk or telephone 0845 601 0174 for information
- Open Universtiy website: www.open.ac.uk or telephone 01908 858585 for general enquiries
- Universty of the Third Age website: www.u3a.org.uk or telephone 0207 8378838

CHAPTER 9

Travel

Is retirement travel different?

Previously travel will have been restricted by the demands of professional life. In retirement the objectives are different. Increased leisure is a wonderful opportunity to extend horizons physically, intellectually and emotionally. Nothing is impossible if you want to do it. Go for it and don't put it off. Being older is no excuse for lazy holidays, rather the reverse. New interests involve you intensely; you become more energetic than when at home. You are freed from the shackles of time and can travel with more convenience and less hassle – and there is no backlog of work to come back to. Whilst health, strength and fitness may work against you, there are ways around this. In compensation, some cultures hold old age in respect and women may avoid the sexual advances of the Latins – unless of course you welcome them!

New interests and activities

We all have different dreams. Will you stick to well-trodden civilisation or make for the back-of-beyond? Will you do-it-yourself or be cosseted by a guide on an organised tour? You could study at a university or a summer school, or maybe you want to go and work on a project in the developing world? Don't think you are too old for activity holidays: if you are fit enough for a few days' walking in Scotland, you will cope with a Himalayan trek, and why shouldn't you go parachute-jumping if you fancy it?

What about wintering in warmer climes when long-term rental of villas and hotel rooms is cheap? Or you could invest in a holiday property bond (this is not time-share). Maybe you are longing to be pampered on a sun-and-sea holiday or a luxury cruise, by all means go, though this is not serious travel. If you are more adventurous, if you want to extend your horizons, then maybe I shall encourage you.

Thorough research and avoiding pitfalls

Looking for new ideas? Seek out "special interest" tour operators. For art, music, wildlife, walking or anything else, you will have enormous choice. Consult the Internet, newspapers or buy magazines specialising in whatever field appeals to you: they contain a vast amount of information with telephone numbers for brochures and websites for you to investigate.

The golden rule is 'read the small print and interpret it'. Not every operator provides the same thing. Competition in the trade is fierce and you really do get what you pay for. The better-quality escorted tours look after you extremely well and attract experts in many fields. A few operators impose an age limit, so check this before you set your heart on something from their brochures, however most leave it to you to decide whether you can cope.

Check what exactly is included. Scheduled flights at convenient hours, or cut-price ones that are the first to be delayed, offer poor back-up and may land you at peripheral airports? Avoid peak periods for travelling and don't go ski-ing during local school holidays. Are all meals and excursions included or only some? Is internal travel by air, coach or railway? The first is a hassle, the second cramped, the third by far the most comfortable, though many tour operators ignore it. Investigate if you will be changing hotels every night which is inconvenient but sometimes unavoidable.

Find out what information you will receive in advance. Reading lists are helpful, as is advice on weather conditions and, especially for Muslim countries, information about local customs (though they seldom tell women always to wear a wedding ring for instance!). If on an escorted tour, ask who goes with you – a tour manager who simply looks after the practicalities or a qualified specialist lecturer who gives talks and encourages discussion? Or are you handed over to local guides who deliver their standard spiel in stilted English? All these details are what you are either paying a higher price for, or economising by doing without them, so read all the small print, ask questions and get clear answers.

Are you a person who makes detailed plans in advance or do you like to let the excitement of a new country take you unawares? In retirement you can afford the latter, for having no preconceived ideas can result in an overwhelming experience you will never forget. Usually though, advance study adds enjoyment and may enable you to include something you particularly want to do. Guidebooks come in different styles, look at several before deciding which is for you. For DIY, read books written for the impecunious young traveller (for example, the *Rough Guide* series, published by Rough Guides, London) – these include more practical information on all aspects of travel. Always ask for senior citizens' concessions for museums and concerts, these vary from country to country. Avoid standing in queues by buying museum tickets in advance from agents in the UK before you travel abroad. You may find that *National Trust* membership cards may be honoured in Commonwealth countries.

How to travel

Travelling by car gives you independence and in North America is almost essential. Taking your own car across the Channel into Europe is easier than ever, with a wide choice of routes. If hiring a car, note that some firms impose an age limit. Don't plan to drive after dark in an unfamiliar car or country, your eyesight may not be as reliable as it used to be and don't be the sole driver unless you are planning to travel short distances.

When leaving the UK by air avoid Heathrow or Gatwick airports if possible. Stansted is as pleasant as any airport can be, with good short-haul and long-haul links and in common with many regional airports is easily accessible from central London. Avoid public transport unless you have minimal baggage. A taxi may be good value even for one person and possibly cheaper than a night in an airport hotel, though sometimes the latter offer free/cheap parking. From central London, a taxi to Heathrow is only marginally more expensive than being dropped at Paddington and taking its rail link. If you are driving yourself to the airport, get parking at half-price by pre-booking (see *Further Information* at the end of this chapter for details). Remember your return – do you really want to drive home after an overnight flight? A chauffeur is a welcome sight.

For long-haul flights consider business class, the difference in the fare between destinations and airlines varies a lot. Discount travel agents offer business and first class bargains as well as economy and will quote you the best prices. The advantage is not free champagne, though this starts the journey well, but space and seating. Pitch of the seat varies between airlines, don't consider anything less than 36 inches. Apart from quicker check-in, lounges and maybe faster luggage delivery, you can generally change your return flight if you turn hippy or wish to stay away for longer, however, for some developing nation airlines, it may not be worth the extra cost and inconvenience.

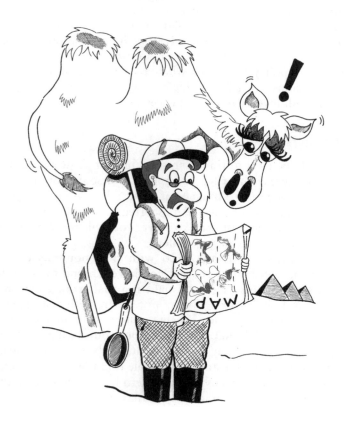

Rail travel at its best is more civilised than flying. In western Europe it is comfortable, reliable and easy to access. Your senior citizen railcard may be valid for railways, buses, boats and ski-lifts. Scenic rail routes in coutries such as South Africa and Australia are incredibly popular and consequently tend to be booked up months in advance.

Luxury cruises are a world of their own, join one if you like expensive dressing-up amongst people with whom you may have little in common and where everything worth doing costs extra. Expedition cruising on the other hand, whether river or sea-going, is quite different in having an educational aim and includes on-board lectures and shore visits. There is huge choice available including history, art, bird-watching, or music to name but a few. It is useful to check the expected number of passengers, since this affects the time it will take to get everyone ashore and back again, and determines whether you meet anyone more than once. A third option is to travel on cargo ships which will often carry a few passengers and present a great opportunity to catch up with leisurely reading. For details of cargo carriers, see the *Further Information* section.

Insurance

Annual insurance cover is far cheaper than for repeated single trips, but insurers are often set against us. Premiums inflate with age and many companies refuse annual cover as early as 65. Fortunately some insurers impose no age limit, but costs vary surprisingly for similar cover, so make sure that you shop around before choosing a policy and check what cover your home insurance offers for personal possessions. Usually a single trip is limited to 45–60 days, and extended visits will involve paying an excess.

Single travellers

You may already be used to travelling solo, but for those facing it for the first time, because of bereavement for example, it is a source of anxiety. To these I would offer the strongest encouragement to start: be courageous, you will not be lonely for more than the first day. An escorted tour with no more than 15–30 participants may be the best way to start, you will meet many people with similar interests in a convivial atmosphere.

As a single traveller, you are faced with the iniquitous choice: a single supplement or sharing. Fine to share if you have a friend to go with, though if you have not shared before, agree to make it a trial arrangement with no hard feelings in case it doesn't work. If you opt to share with a stranger – on board ships this is expensive to avoid – agents will try to match you up. You may request non-smoking and English-speaking but you can hardly demand a non-snorer! The alternative is to pay a supplement, but be sure it is worth it. Are you getting single occupancy of a standard double room or a small back room with no view? As a rough rule, if staying in modern hotels you can get the former, if in the "traditional inns of character" you may get the latter. Note what meals are included, no-one minds scavenging lunch but dining alone in the evening is not much fun and until you get to know your fellow travellers, you may unintentionally be left out.

Health and fitness

Let's be honest, as we age we are losing some of our own strength, stamina, balance and eyesight and are less tolerant of heat and cold. Minor illnesses are more upsetting as we grow older, and eventually we face the frailties of old age.

Travel as lightly as possible. Use trolley suitcases, as you can often find ramps. For hand baggage take a small rucksack, weight feels less when carried on the shoulders and arms are free for holding rails or a walking stick. Don't think a stick ages you, even the young use them nowadays and they do help on rough surfaces. If you are frail or disabled do not despair, porters and wheelchairs can be ordered in advance, though some historic buildings may be out of reach. Try the charity "Holiday Care" for advice and information on travel with a wheelchair (see *Further Information* at the end of this chapter for details). If you are travelling in Asia, off the beaten track, ask yourself if your joints cope with very basic squatting loos? (And ladies, if you wear a long loose skirt you can urinate almost anywhere as discreetly as men can!)

When packing, don't ask "might I need this?" but "can I possibly do without it?" Do you need more shoes than one comfortable pair for daytime and one smarter pair for evenings? Dress in layers, thin trousers plus long-johns for when it turns cold saves taking thick ones. The same principle applies with tops, and for women I would advise a pair of black trousers with a variety of tops will see us anywhere from a country walk to the opera. Don't take more of anything than you need: decant creams into small jars and discard packaging. Take reading matter to throw or give away, thus creating space as you travel. Don't be tempted to buy souvenirs, your house is full of everything you need and agree with your family not to bring presents back.

Take any regular drugs you use, plus a pack for accidents and emergencies. If hospital standards are doubtful and HIV is prevalent, take a sealed pack including syringes and intravenous delivery set. Reduce the risk of deep-vein-thrombosis during flights in particular by wearing elastic stockings, and for long journeys in general by taking a low-dose aspirin (unless you have a contraindication). Ensure that you get up-to-date information from a travel clinic or the Department of Health about immunisations and prophylactic regimes which change continually (see *Further Information* at the end of this chapter for details). For protection against malaria, don't rely only on drugs, avoid bites by wearing cover-up garments, protect skin with an insect repellent such as deet, try to stay indoors after dark and sleep under a mosquito net if possible.

Heed the advice you give patients about sensible eating. Where water safety is dubious, don't trust it, even luxury hotels may be unreliable. Buy bottled water in large containers from the supermarket rather than the hotel fridge and check that the cap seal is unbroken. In primitive conditions be independent and safe by taking a kettle for boiling, or a small filter and iodine drops (plus vitamin C tablets to remove the taste). Be prudent about pre-cooked or raw food, ice-cream and ice cubes in drinks. Make all this a habit, without being obsessional, and you can remain healthy anywhere, I've done it many times.

Finally…
Be enterprising, and don't believe anything is closed to you: exercise your body, mind and spirit, and the world is yours. I wish you at least as much reward and enjoyment in your travels as I am still having after 18 years of retirement.

AKA

Further information

- *BMA Members Guide to Working Abroad* (Feb 2001). Telephone: 020 7385 6231
- Holiday Property Bond. Telephone: 01638 660066; website: www.hpb.co.uk
- BAA – for information about British airports, parking, flight information. Website: www.baa.co.uk
- The Air Transport Users Council produces a booklet for passengers with special needs called *Flight Plan*. The booklet can be obtained from: Air Transport Users Council, CAA House, 45–58 Kingsway, London WC2B 6TE. Telephone: 020 7240 6061 (between 2 pm–5 pm)
- Heathrow Travel Care (a Heathrow based charity) Room 1308, Queens' Building, Heathrow Airport, Hounslow, Middlesex TW6 IBZ. Telephone: 020 8745 7495
- Tripscope – transport information service for people with impaired mobility The Vassall Centre, Gill Avenue, Bristol, BS16 2QQ Telephone/textphone: 08457 58 56 51 or e-mail: tripscope@cableinet.co.uk
- Senior Railcard, ATOC Ltd, Third Floor, 40 Bernard Street, London WC1N 1BY. Website: www.senior-railcard.co.uk
- American Express, local branches.
- For details of freighter passenger services contact: The Cruise People Ltd, Telephone: 020 7723 2450; website: members.aol.com/CruiseAZ/freighters.htm
- Trailfinders – largest UK independent travel company. Telephone: 020 7938 3444 or see local branches; website: www.trailfinders.com
- Insurers giving annual cover without age limit: Age Concern – Telephone: 0800 169 2700; website: www.ageconcern.org.uk Argos Travel Insurance – Telephone: 0800 013 6622 Green Flag – Telephone: 0800 328 8755; website: www.greenflag.co.uk NatWest – Telephone: 0800 505050; website: www.natwest.com Options Travel Insurance – Telephone: 0870 876 7878 Woolwich Travel Insurance – Telephone: 0870 602 0542; website: www.woolwich.co.uk

- Holiday Care – information packs for elderly and less mobile travellers. 2nd floor, Imperial Buildings, Victoria Rd, Horley, Surrey, RH6 7PZ. Telephone: 01293 774535; website: www.holidaycare.org.uk
- Homeway medical. Telephone: 01980 626361; e-mail: travelwithcare@homeway.co.uk
- YHA Adventure Shops, for local branches contact Customer Services: 0870 870 8808; website: www.yha.org.uk. Free booklet '*Travellers' Companion*'.

Health advice for travellers:
- British Airways travel clinics. Website: www.britishairways.com/travelclinics/
  156 Regent Street, London W1B 5LB. Walk-in service Mon–Fri: 09.30 am–5.15 pm, Sat: 10 am–4 pm. Or appointments available Mon–Fri by telephone: 020 7439 9584
  101 Cheapside, London EC2V 6DT. Telephone: 020 7606 2977 to make an appointment
- Department of Health. Telephone: 0800 555 777; website: www.doh.gov.uk/traveladvice
- Malaria reference laboratory. Telephone: 09065 508 908; website: www.malaria-reference.co.uk
- Medical Advisory Services for Travellers Abroad (MASTA), based at the London School of Hygiene and Tropical Medicine. Travellers' Health Line: 0906 8224100; website: www.masta.org
- Foreign and Commonwealth Office, Travel Advice Unit, Consular Division, Old Admiralty Building, London SW1A 2PA. Advice line: 020 7008 0232/0233 or fax: 020 7008 0155; website: www.fco.gov.uk/travel/

(information correct at May 2002)

CHAPTER 10

Returning to old interests

It is hardly surprising that so many doctors have taken up painting and sculpture as a hobby. Drawing and modelling call for coordination of hand and eye, and a sound knowledge of anatomy helps in life drawing and portraiture. Most doctor-artists have been content to make art their hobby, but some of these have been to a very high standard. Lord Lister made beautiful water-colour paintings of the microbes he saw through his father's invention, the achromatic microscope, sometimes using the *camera lucida*. Sir Henry Thompson, the pioneer of litholopaxy for calculi in the bladder, regularly exhibited at the Royal Academy. The father of plastic surgery Sir Harold Gillies was said to be as expert with the fly-rod and the paintbrush as he was with the knife and held regular exhibitions of his work. Sir Henry Souttar, the pioneer heart surgeon, was an unusual draughtsman who illustrated his own textbooks and was a talented cartoonist. Some went so far as to forsake medicine for art: Henry Tonks who had trained as a surgeon under Treves left surgery to teach at the Slade, where Augustus John was among his pupils.

At the BMA meeting in Bournemouth in 1934 a successful art exhibition was held and the idea of forming a Medical Art Society was first mooted. The leading lights were Sir Leonard Hill, the celebrated physiologist, Charles Pannett, Geoffrey Bourne, Sir Harold Gillies and Norman Silvester. The society, which is now based at the Royal Society of Medicine in London, holds annual exhibitions which are well attended, and organizes painting expeditions and life-drawing sessions. It is open to doctors and dentists, and it encourages students and spouses to exhibit at the annual exhibition. (Details of membership may be obtained from the Royal Society of Medicine.)

Most of us have been painting or sculpting all our lives, and many of us share the naughty habit of doodling on committee papers. (The doodles bring back the occasion if not the agenda in the way that no notes can do.) While attending scientific meetings overseas the odd little sketch made on a visit can be much more interesting than any number of colour photographs. For people like this retirement changes nothing, it just gives more time to indulge a life-long hobby. This article is not for them; it is for the many others who enjoyed painting and drawing at school, but gave it up under the growing pressures of the curriculum, the need to pass endless professional examinations, daily clinical commitments and the calls of home and family. The paints were put on one side, or given to the children. The sack of clay has long ago dried up. In retirement, the idea occurs to them, that it might be fun to start again. But how?

I believe that the first step is to join a congenial art group. You will find that every group includes people with a wide range of skills, tastes and ability and it does not matter if they are more or less experienced, what matters most is that they should be good company. There are bound to be several such groups in your neighbourhood, and evening classes are provided by most local authorities. The monthly art journals and the glossies from the Tate and the Royal Academy give details of these, and of course, you could do a lot worse than to join the Medical Art Society.

Teachers vary too: not everyone will find the same person equally helpful, but for even the most experienced amateur a teacher can be a stimulus and a help; even Olympic sportsmen continue to use the services of a professional coach. Apart from anything else the professional will advise you on basic matters of technique: what paints to use, how to prepare canvas, what brushes to use, and how to keep them clean. There are also a number of technical tricks which no book can teach; how to lay a wash in water colour, how to use glazes in oils and so on.

Painting

When the weather is good there is nothing (to my mind) more agreeable than to go out with an old friend, and try to paint *en plein air*. It may help to take one or two photographs so that you can work on the painting later on at home, though I find photographs in general of limited help; the colours never seem right. Painting is thirsty work, and a picnic certainly helps the muse. Above everything it should be fun, and not taken seriously.

When the weather is foul, you can work on your old sketches indoors, or try to paint a still life, e.g. a group of pots, fruit or flowers. Or you can find someone patient enough to sit for portrait, which of all forms of painting is one that I personally find most interesting and challenging.

Watercolours

There is no end to the different media you can use. One tends to think first of watercolour because the materials are cheap and portable, but it is the least forgiving and allows little room for making mistakes. Some have unhappy memories of our childhood paint boxes, with their innumerable pans which all looked so bright in the box, but somehow turned to mud on the paper. Now that you are grown up treat yourself to the best quality paints. You will find that the colours stay clear and bright. You do not need many but you do need good ones. My own little box contains burnt umber, aquamarine, coerulean blue, sap green, scarlet, alizarin, Indian red, chrome yellow, yellow ochre and cadmium yellow. I use solid paints: others prefer tubes.

Your brush should be able to hold a lot of water, and come to a fine point. You only need one or two, so it is sensible to get a good one, and the kind whose handle forms a hollow protective case will prevent the brush being ruined by being bent over.

There are many different kinds of paper for watercolours. Thin paper curls up when wet. You can go to all the trouble of sticking it onto a board, but it is really easier to buy good thick paper: if you get paper with a fairly coarse grain a wash of aquamarine or burnt umber collects in the little dimples in the most attractive way.

Amateurs usually set out to paint classical English watercolours using clean washes and only the lightest underdrawing in pencil, but a much easier technique is that of line-and-wash. The secret here is to use India Ink. Once it has dried it will not run when a wash of watercolour is laid over it. I carry with me two of the architects' 'Rotring' pens, with 0.35 and 0.5 mm nibs. The only snag about them is that they clog up and every two or three weeks need to be washed out with warm water and a little washing-up liquid.

It is very easy to ruin a promising watercolour, and you must harden yourself to the need to be brutal, throw it away and start all over again. For the same reason there is no need to finish the painting all at one go: a sketch made in the open air can always be finished at home, or repeated using more (and cleaner) water.

Pastels

Painting with pastels is quite a different experience. There are a large number of different types, some softer than others, and all of them apt to engender a kind of grey dust which gets everywhere. The finished painting is easily smudged and spoilt, and there is a purist school of thought which insists that the pastels should not be fixed because the fixative will spoil the colour. I do not think this is true with modern fixatives, and was interested to learn at a recent exhibition that Degas himself thought nothing of fixing his pastels, working over them again, until he had built up quite a considerable thickness. Nobody can accuse his colours of being dull. One of the advantages of pastel is that they are easy to carry about. Again, the beginner is apt to be seduced by enormous boxes containing every shade and colour. In practice they can be mixed on the paper or added on top of each other so that you do not need a huge range. It is more important to get good ones with clear, bright colours.

Oils

One of the great advantages of painting in oils is that if you make a mistake it is easy to paint over it, or scrape it off and start again. With oil paints, again, it pays to get good ones, and keep a limited palette. I use the same colours I have listed for watercolour, only in addition you need white. For brushes you can choose between round and flat ones, and you do not need a huge number and you do not need to buy the most expensive. So long as you clean them at the end of the day, using soap and water or washing-up liquid, they will last indefinitely, but if you let them harden you may as well throw them away. You can paint on almost any surface so long as it is adequately primed with acrylic, but there is something agreeable about canvas. I used to stretch my own, but ready-made canvases are almost as cheap, and a good deal more convenient.

There are as many different ways of using oil paint as there are artists. The paint can be diluted with white spirit and used in thin transparent 'washes', or you can put it on thick, straight out of the tube. The range of effects you can produce are never-ending, and each painting becomes a different experiment.

Sculpture

Carving in stone or wood appeals to many of us, but it is messy, and you really need somewhere where you can create a lot of noise and dust. Modelling on the other hand can be done almost anywhere, with minimum mess. Clay is the classical medium, but it must be kept moist or it will dry out and crack away from the armature, and for this reason many of my friends use modelling wax. I have come to prefer plasticine or the similar material called "Lewis's Newplast", which handles like clay, but does not dry up and crack.

The steps of making a sculpture are no different today than they were in the time of Benevenuto Cellini. You begin with an armature, for which most people use the flexible aluminium extrusion which is attached to a wooden post. This is then covered over with tape or string, to give the clay something to stick on to. Then one builds up the figure using progressively smaller lumps until the required form is achieved. Tiranti's, the sculptor's supply shop in Warren Street, London has all the necessary materials, and a good range of very practical manuals which show you how to construct an armature.

If you want to keep your sculpture it has to be cast. The traditional material for a cast is plaster of Paris, but using this is messy work: the plaster gets everywhere and it is necessary to take special care not to let any get into the drains or you will have an expensive blockage to put right. Tiranti's will put you in touch with young sculptors who will do your casting for you for a small fee.

By putting powdered metal into a gel coat one can make a polyester resin cast that can look exactly like a genuine bronze, and with skill it is possible to produce a very similar range of patination. You will see many such resin sculptures in exhibitions, often referred to as 'cold-cast bronze'. The technique is not difficult to master, although the resin smells, and final trimming of the work with a powder-sander is very dusty. If you intend to keep your sculpture out of doors there is a risk of deterioration of the resin surface. On the other hand if you made a particularly satisfying sculpture there is nothing nicer than a genuine bronze, but of course this calls for the expertise of a bronze founder, and it is costly, not least because bronze itself is valuable. Bronze founders advertise in the art journals. Alternatively, Tiranti's also have a wide selection of handbooks covering the use of clay and the making of casts in plaster, *ciment fondu* and fibreglass.

One of the most unexpected delights that flow from painting or sculpting as a hobby is that it makes a visit to an exhibition or a gallery ten times more interesting. One is constantly struck by some clever trick, some solution to a vexing problem, some odd juxtaposition of colours which seems worth imitating. Most of us have dissected too many dogfish to be interested in shark formalin, or to want to cross the road to see yet another grubby crumpled bed, but now that you are retired, you will have plenty of time to visit exhibitions and galleries, and the more you do yourself, the more you will enjoy them.

JPB

Further information

- Medical Art Society, Royal Society of Medicine, 1 Wimpole Street, London W1G 0AE; telephone: 020 7290 3948; website: www.rsm.ac.uk/social/arts.htm#medicalarts
- Alec Tiranti Ltd, 27 Warren Street, London W1T 5NB. Telephone: 020 7636 8565 or fax: 020 7636 8565; website: www.tiranti.co.uk

CHAPTER 11

History, writing and editing

Doctors face the prospect of retirement in many different ways. Some, on retiring from the NHS, find clinical practice so enjoyable that they undertake locum appointments or private practice; some become increasingly involved in national and international committee work in colleges, faculties and other organisations; others turn their backs on medicine and grow roses, play golf or indulge in a variety of absorbing leisure pursuits; yet others revive cultural interests long neglected in a busy professional career, such as music and the arts; there are even some who undertake university courses in topics such as archaeology, philosophy or the history of art.

My experience

For myself, I can justly claim to have retired three times. My appointment in Newcastle upon Tyne was a so-called "A+B" appointment, with five NHS sessions as a consultant neurologist and six university sessions as professor of neurology (and, for ten years, dean of medicine). When I moved to become warden of Green College in Oxford, I retired from my NHS appointment and became a whole-time university employee. At the same time, I was president of the General Medical Council, but retired under the council's rules from that post after seven years in 1989, just six months before my retirement from the wardenship of Green College when the age limit became effective. Even then, as I had negotiated on moving to Oxford honorary clinical contracts with Oxford District and Region, I continued to do limited teaching and to see a few patients until in 1992, shortly after my 70th birthday, I received a letter from the Oxfordshire Health Authority pointing out that now I had reached that age, my honorary clinical contract had expired and I could visit the hospital for social reasons but could use no clinical facilities. In the event, having become a life peer in the Birthday Honours List of 1989, I soon found myself heavily involved in the work of the House of Lords as a cross-bencher and have remained active in promoting the interests of medicine, science and education in the Upper House ever since.

Hence, although I can justly claim throughout my working life to have had many activities to occupy my mind, I confess that on the day after my retirement from Green College I sat in my study at 13 Norham Gardens (Sir William Osler's old home) realising for the first time that I did not have to go to work and wondering just how I was going to make the best use of my time. It was then that I decided that a long-established interested in medical history, never significantly indulged because of the pressure of other commitments, would be something in which I would take an increasing interest. I also knew that writing and editing would be other commitments that I would happily continue to undertake.

History

In my medical student days in Newcastle upon Tyne, I was introduced by the late Sir James Spence, professor of child health, to the writings of Sir William Osler, which I then read avidly. I found them compelling and inspiring to such an extent that the first paper I wrote in the Durham University Students' Medical Gazette in 1943 was entitled *A great physician* and was based upon the life of Osler. William Osler was born in Bond Head, Ontario, the son of an Anglican clergyman who had emigrated to Canada in response to a call for missionaries. He subsequently went to school in Dundas, Ontario, before studying medicine at McGill University, where he later became professor of medicine, before moving consecutively to Philadelphia (the University of Pennsylvania) and then to Johns Hopkins Hospital, Baltimore, where he was the Foundation professor of medicine. He was a great bibliophile with a love of medical history, but it is his writings that have assured for him a secure reputation as one of the greatest physicians of all time. Anyone who has read his *Aequanimitas and Other Essays to Medical Students and Other Health Professionals*, his *An Alabama Student and Other Essays* or *Counsels and Ideals* cannot help but be affected, as I was, by his approach to medical practice and the inspirational nature of his teaching, as well as by his love of books and his love of history. All too often, he pointed out to the enquiring physician that some of what he or she may have thought to be flashes of inspiration had previously been recognised by physicians of yesteryear. Cushing's *Life of Osler* must surely be one of the greatest biographies ever written. Even now, when Osler societies flourish in many countries across the world including Canada, the United States, the United Kingdom and Japan, to name but four, Osler's life and work continue to inspire; a recently-published new biography entitled *William Osler: A Life in Medicine* by Michael Bliss is yet another admirable publication. Tentatively, even now, I continue to collect material about the history of 20th century neurology and may yet decide to publish something on this topic.

For any doctor now retired or about to retire, admirable reference sources are available in the many textbooks of medical history (Castiglione's is a favourite of mine), in relevant journals such as the *Journal of Medical Biography* (JMB), and in the voluminous libraries and archives of the medical Royal Colleges, the Royal Society of Medicine, and the Wellcome Trust's History of Medicine Library. Why not aim to publish a paper in the JMB? Even if, for linguistic reasons or for difficulty of access, it may not be possible invariably to consult original sources, it is often fruitful to collate and analyse information from previous publications in a manner not previously achieved.

Writing

Since my schooldays, I have loved the English language, have tried to appreciate its more complex nuances and have enjoyed manipulating words, even though in writing, as in many other activities, I sometimes feel that I have probably lacked originality and flair. Writing, however, has usually come easily although, like everyone who puts pen to paper, I have suffered intermittently from those curious mental blocks when one stares either at a blank sheet of paper, at a silent dictating machine or, nowadays, at a word processor, finding that the words simply fail to flow. Sometimes they have, however, flowed more readily, no doubt with consequential prolixity. Nevertheless, my love of, and enjoyment in, language has always made me impatient and intolerant of carelessness in its usage and in grammatical construction. Misspelling by the highly intelligent I can tolerate, accepting that this may be a specific, if minor, learning defect which is difficult to overcome, as in the case, it is said, of Dr Samuel Johnson and Edgar Allen Poe. Having learned Latin at school, I have been compelled to tolerate 'forums' rather than 'fora', but nevertheless cringe when I see a split infinitive or when someone, as is usual nowadays, talks about 'different to' rather than 'different from'. I cannot avoid a sense of surprise on learning that expensively educated and outstandingly intelligent young people now lack the grammatical

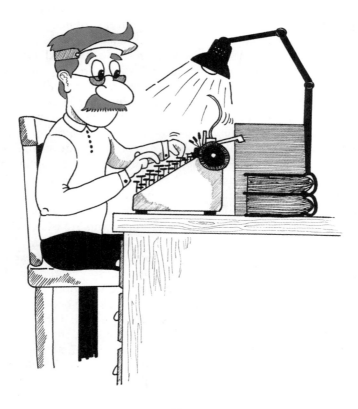

knowledge which was drummed into us all in my schooldays. Many are unable to distinguish between a simile and a metaphor, fail to appreciate the proper use of adverbs and do not recognise that the word "prior" should only be used as an adjective. And the incorrect use of "I" and "me" ("she talked to him and I") or the preposition coming at the end of a sentence ("this was something I was not aware of") continue to irritate. Is the battle of correct English usage irrevocably lost?

I first took an interest in writing in school and produced a duplicated newspaper, as well as writing for the school magazine. Later, during my medical student days, after writing the article on William Osler to which I have already referred, I wrote another on *Thomas Sydenham, the English Hippocrates*, but subsequently became so embroiled in medical matters that I turned to medical writing, publishing a paper in *The Lancet* while still a house officer on the physical basis of continuous intravenous infusions. After my army service, when I returned to Newcastle as a medical registrar, I embarked upon an extensive study of subarachnoid haemorrhage which led to my MD thesis and this was subsequently published in a monograph by E & S Livingstone, as later was a book on *Polymyositis* written jointly with my friend and mentor, Professor Raymond Adams of Boston, where I spent a year in the Massachusetts General Hospital from 1953 to 1954.

The writing bug continued to be an important part of my life in publishing the results of my research into neuromuscular disease over the next 20 years, but I was also pleased to be invited to write a short textbook of neurology (*Essentials of Neurology*, first published by Pitman and subsequently going to six editions), followed by *Disorders of Voluntary Muscle* (Churchill and later Churchill Livingstone), a multi-author text which again I edited through some six editions. The travails of multi-authorship are well known to many writers and editors, and these were subsequently highlighted when, after moving from Newcastle to Oxford in 1983, I was asked by Oxford University Press to take on the senior editorship of *The Oxford Companion to Medicine*, originally conceived by Professor Paul Beeson and Sir Ronald Bodley Scott. Preparation and production of this encyclopaedic two-volume work was incredibly demanding and time-consuming, but nevertheless functioned as a remarkable educational tool as I learned a great deal from reading and editing all of the short or more lengthy contributions. Human nature being what it is, there are some authors who are very prompt in submitting manuscripts and others who are exceptionally tardy and who need more than encouragement in order to produce. Frantic and increasingly irate letters and telephone calls usually, in my experience, solve the problem, but almost invariably I found, in *Disorders of Voluntary Muscle* and in *The Oxford Companion to Medicine*, a twelve-month spread between receiving the first and the last contributions. Only on two occasions can I recall being compelled to discard authors because of non-compliance.

Yet another challenge arose in 1966 following the death of the great neurologist, Lord Brain, when his son and widow invited me to revise his classical text, *Diseases of the Nervous System*, which had been one of the most successful textbooks of neurology ever written. The seventh edition was a hybrid, partly revised by Lord Brain before his death and partly by myself, but the eighth (published in 1977) was entirely my own, as was the ninth, which appeared in 1985. By that time, however, it became clear that advances in neurology were so great that it was no longer possible, in my view, to produce a comprehensive textbook on neurology by a single author; hence, the tenth edition, published in 1993, was a multi-author volume under my editorship. It is good to know that *Disorders of Voluntary Muscle* and *The Oxford Medical Companion* are now being published under new editors, as I felt in 1996, when in my mid-seventies, that the time had come for me to hand over the reins.

Editing

Inevitably, when one achieves senior status in neurology, one is approached about editing journals. Without personal recompense, I edited the *Journal of the Neurological Sciences* from 1966 to 1977; this was the official journal of the World Federation of Neurology. Probably I was naïve, but I certainly had not appreciated that many journal editors in the USA and subsequently in the UK were remunerated for their efforts. I, with my long-serving secretary, Rosemary Allan, handled all the papers submitted from many parts of the world and we were often compelled virtually to rewrite, for example, those submitted in English by colleagues from Japan and elsewhere. The task was arduous, involving many late hours and early mornings, but it was nevertheless fruitful, though I was happy to hand over the reins to Professor WB (Bryan) Matthews in 1977 (my good friend, Bryan, sadly died in July 2001). My subsequent editorship of *Current Opinion in Neurology* was equally fruitful but much less demanding.

One of the problems I found throughout in editorial work was that of correcting infelicities of phrasing, as well as grammatical and typographical errors which abounded in many of the manuscripts which I had to consider over the years. Being somewhat obsessional, I find it distressing that so many authors submit manuscripts which have been carelessly written and poorly prepared; by the time I had finished editing many of them, the pages were strewn with my corrections and comments. Can authors not be persuaded to read carefully and correct their effusions? Much the same problems were also encountered repeatedly in proof correction as a result of careless typesetting in the course of production. I well recall one page of *The Oxford Companion to Medicine* typeset in the headquarters of the Oxford University Press, in which I was required to make 68 proof corrections.

The reader may reasonably ask "Is it all worthwhile?" Financially, the answer must certainly be "No", as even successful medical textbooks generate very little in the way of income and the rewards are invariably out of proportion to the amount of work involved. In making this comment, I must exclude from consideration my more recent responsibilities in editing books in the *International Congress and Symposium Series* for the Royal Society of Medicine. Here, too, many of the manuscripts require substantial modification, not least in relation to the scientific data presented, but also in respect of grammatical and typographical errors and infelicities of phrasing. I believe that the rewards for this work are entirely reasonable and I hope to continue with this task for some time to come. But I cannot resist a sense of astonishment when I find that a manuscript, having already been edited by a distinguished scientific editor, contains surprising errors. In one such, for example, the scientific editor had gone through the entire manuscript changing 'these data are' to 'this data is', and yet another such editor persisted in writing 'this phenomena is'. These are but two of many examples I could readily quote which make me feel that much greater attention to grammatical construction in our beautiful language is needed in our schools. Another problem is the vanishing adverb, when one hears leading golfers say, for example, "I played solid"!

Conclusions

As in my advancing years I now struggle manfully with word processing, e-mails and other computer mysteries, I recognise that the whole area of writing and publishing has been transformed. It is a far cry from the time when I used to dictate scientific papers on to a tape so that Rosemary could transcribe the first draft, as indeed I did in writing my autobiography, *The Spice of Life*, published by the Royal Society of Medicine and Heinemann in 1993. I can only say that to continue to be involved in a limited amount of writing and a considerable amount of editing in my retirement has been fruitful and rewarding and I can commend to any doctor facing retirement the idea of turning to a study of medical history, which so illumines modern-day clinical practice, and to the exciting use, if not of the pen or typewriter, then of the computer.

JW

CHAPTER 12

Computing

Many of you will have completed your work careers having had little contact with personal computers (PCs), however there is no excuse for this continuing into retirement. A computer has much to offer the active individual, and can prove to be both a stimulating new hobby and a way of developing and maintaining new interests.

This chapter provides a brief introduction to the role a PC can play in your life, some basic information on buying a PC, and guidance on sources of training and advice. Although concentrating on PCs, many of the comments are relevant to Apple Macintosh computers.

Why should I bother with a PC?

Some weeks before this was written, I was on the telephone to a helpline operative, trying to fathom out why my infernal machine (a.k.a. PC) was misbehaving, just when I needed it most. After ten minutes or so of conversation and repeated trials and errors with ultimate success, he asked me my year of birth, and when I told him it was 1925 he sounded totally astonished that such an elderly gent should be computer literate. The young tend to regard modern technology as their province, but it need not be so. If you have a logical mind and the discipline and patience that comes with age, you may find yourself much less disadvantaged than you think. Technical advances have made the use of computers appreciably easier and more reliable than in earlier days.

However, those of us well advanced in the seven ages, who have already chanced our arms with computers, may well need encouragement to explore their virtues in greater depth, which, it has to be said, have from time to time been thought to be outweighed by their vices. Having said that, remembering that computers are nothing more than sophisticated tools, they pose a challenge to the user. Once you learn what can be done and what cannot be done (at least for the time being), which leads to the knowledge of what to do, and, more importantly, what not to do, the rewards are impressive.

At a recent meeting of the Medico-Legal Society, Professor TBL Kirkwood indicated how exercise would slow down the degeneration of muscle cell DNA. When asked whether mental exercise would do the same for the cerebral neurones, he was quite encouraging in his response. Whatever may be the faults of computers, their use certainly stimulates the Betz cells. Even simple games like FreeCell (provided with Windows) challenge observation and strategy. Better still, there are programmes which enable you to sit down with a virtual trio and play bridge, and your partner at the virtual table cannot complain about your poor bidding.

To the uninitiated, computers may seem conspicuous by their potential ability to confuse, irritate and frighten. Advancing years have been a prominent excuse for avoiding having anything to do with them. The result is that the rewards from successfully using these remarkable tools and their ever-developing technology are never experienced. There is so much to enjoy for relatively little cost, and to forgo these advantages by dint of an archetypal fear born out of the unknown would be a great shame.

There are three main areas in which the computer comes into its own. Together with a colour printer it becomes a tool which replaces a typewriter, your filing system and even the local photography and print shop – it is astonishingly effective. It saves money too, as you can produce your own letterheads, visiting cards, birthday cards, and a whole host of items of considerable quality which you would normally purchase from time to time. Your photo albums are also in danger of becoming extinct. Digital photography enables you to take a photo, process it with improvements if you wish, then print it out or send it as an email within moments of clicking the button on the camera. There are several programmes available which allow you to screen slide shows with the greatest of ease.

The second area is communication. With the assistance of a modem (a device that may be inside your computer or external to it) and your telephone line, you may now contact anyone, anywhere in the world, in seconds, by email, and all for the cost of a local telephone call. You may send text and graphics, so photos and even videoclips can be with your far flung relatives and friends in a flash. Voice transmission is also possible, and cheap telephone calls via the Internet are becoming more viable every day. Be warned, though, that email is about as private as if you were transmitting from the top of Mount Everest. It is also possible to send and receive faxes via your PC either directly through phone lines, or, more recently, via the net.

Finally as a source of information it is unsurpassed. What was originally dubbed the Superhighway is now well established as the Internet, the World Wide Web or simply "the net". Every morning I connect to the net and read not only several English newspapers, but also others from the USA or elsewhere, depending on what's happening in the world. Learning how to use, or "surf", the net is not difficult – there are numerous magazines available in newsagents and RSM Press, for example, has produced several excellent books about the Internet which are extremely helpful. The net is a mine of information on any subject you care to consider. Once accessed, you can print the information out for safe keeping or download it to your PC for future use.

Another bonus is the opportunity to conduct my banking via the net. This means I can maintain and manipulate my accounts, pay various bills, set up direct debits etc, at any time day or night without leaving my desk. I also have no hesitation in buying books, CDs, DVDs and other items such as travel or concert tickets over the net. The systems seem to be secure when so designated, and so far I have not run into trouble.

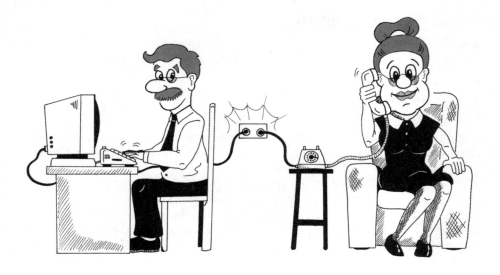

What do I need to do to get connected to the Internet?

You will have to choose an Internet Service Provider (ISP) and choosing the right ISP is important, particularly if you live a fair way from the telephone exchange. The quality of data transmission over telephone lines varies inversely with the length of the line. British Telecom guarantees voice transmission over its lines, but not data. Your ISP provides the "server" with which your computer will communicate, and not all servers can cope with the extra efficiency that distant lines require. You will need to try them out, and since competition is great, most will offer free trials. There are ISPs that provide free services, so all you have to pay for are the telephone calls. Some offer "unmetered access," which may involve you paying a lump sum up front or a monthly subscription which covers the entire cost. See what is on offer and experiment, but do not commit yourself to a long-term contract until you are quite sure that the system works to your satisfaction. If you want to compare a number of ISPs then the *Internet Magazine* publishes a monthly listing of ISPs. Don't worry that connecting to the net will require specialist skills: as Robert Kiley says in *The Patient's Internet Handbook* (RSM Press) "Anyone who can install a computer game or piece of office software has the necessary skills to connect a computer to the Internet".

There is also an extensive library of books available to help you not only with the Windows operating system itself but with individual programmes that you may decide to install. In any case, all the best programmes incorporate help files which should be able to answer questions that confront you, and if these are inadequate, there is always more information on the net.

ND

Buying your first computer

Whether you are buying your first computer or upgrading to a newer model, I'm sure that you will have three objectives in mind, to buy a machine that:

- meets your needs
- is easy to use and reliable
- doesn't cost too much.

With the increase in computing power over the last few years it should be relatively easy to find the right specification PC which will meet all your needs, now and at least for a few years to come. It is important however to acknowledge that PCs, like cars, are continuously superseded by newer, better and faster models. However, like cars, last year's model will still work adequately. There are bargains available if you are not set upon the latest model, although it is particularly important to consider what you will be using it for before you make your choice, especially if you plan to use particular software or carry out certain tasks such as graphics processing. Here are some of the key areas where you will need to make sure that what's on offer actually meets your requirements:

PC specification

Generally speaking any PC on sale in the high street or via mail order should be able to handle all the things that you will throw at it. However, you should note that if you are planning to use your computer to store a large number of digital images you should pay particular attention to disk space, and if you want to be able to play games (whether for you or for grandchildren) then RAM and video memory are the most important components.

As a minimum you should be looking for a PC with a processor speed of at least 1000 megahertz (MHz) also referred to as 1 gigahertz (1GHz), and it is already very common to see speeds of 1.5 or 2 GHz on the high street. The second most important consideration is the amount of working memory, known as RAM – certainly don't settle for less than 256 MB (megabytes), but if you can afford it, 512 MB is probably a good investment – particularly for playing games (you will also need a good amount of video memory, say 32 MB). Your next priority is disk storage space; this shouldn't be a problem as most machines seem to come with 20 GB or even 40 GB (gigabytes) and this should be more than adequate for most users (even for those storing digital images). But if you can get more for a reasonable price you will probably end up using it, since computers are like attics and garages and soon fill up, not with junk but with potentially useful information! Don't forget you will need a printer, and since colour ink-jet printers are now quite cheap it's well worth opting for one. You may find that you are offered a printer, scanner or digital camera as part of a "package": this is often a good way to get a good deal, but do be sure that the devices offered will meet your needs.

Software

The majority of new PCs will come with a fairly comprehensive collection of software, which should meet (almost) all of your needs. You should find that the PC comes with the Microsoft Windows XP (short for the Windows Experience) operating system (introduced in October 2001), and this has a standard number of features which make digital photography, accessing music files, and using your computer to communicate with others over the Internet much easier. It also has the capacity to "repair" itself when software problems occur, which should make life easier as well. The operating system contains all the intelligence your computer needs to communicate with the hardware and other software packages that you use, and now also includes useful pieces of software such as *Internet Explorer* and email software, as well as other utilities.

There really isn't a choice when it comes to the most important software package – you will need an '*Office*' suite, which includes word processing, spreadsheets, databases and presentation software, and it seems that the world's choice is *Microsoft Office*. This package has almost all of the so-called 'productivity' software that you will need and again the latest version is called *XP*. Within *Windows* and *Office XP* you should have all the software you need to write letters, manage your finances, store and organise data, including pictures video and music. You will be able to connect to the Internet (via your ISP), look at websites and send email. With an additional package such as Microsoft *Publisher* you will also be able to produce a range of more sophisticated printed materials including business cards, headed paper, flyers and posters. It is worth noting that *Office* is a very expensive piece of software with a full retail price of over £400 – if you buy a new PC make sure that it is included in the price. It shouldn't add a lot to the total cost and the investment will certainly pay off in the future.

You may find that Microsoft *Works Suite* is on offer, and whilst this doesn't have the full functionality of *Office*, it probably has everything that the home (or even small business) user will need. At the time of writing the latest version, *Works Suite 2001*, includes: *Word 2000*, spreadsheet, database, calendar, address book and some other general software including a publishing package.

Beyond these "basics" there is a whole world of software out there for you to add to your PC, ranging from games, through very useful packages such as route planning software, to a whole host of add-ons which can keep you occupied for hours. As always with a computer the golden rule is to check that the specification of your PC (processor type/speed, RAM and hard disk capacity) meets the requirements of the package before you buy!

Upgrades

Having read all this, you may well feel that your computer will meet all your needs for the future and beyond! However, it is a fact of life in the PC world that at some point an upgrade will be needed. Certainly it is difficult to forecast exactly what the requirements of future versions of *Windows* and *Office* will be, and who knows what new technology or application is waiting out there.

However, if you buy wisely this shouldn't be a problem. We have already established that PCs sold today should have plenty of capacity to do the job you have in mind – what they should also have is the capacity to be upgraded. If you buy from a reputable manufacturer or retailer, the PC should have the ability to take extra memory and even to have some components like the video card replaced if your needs change. It is certainly worthwhile asking the salesperson if there are spare sockets for additional RAM, and how many free slots there are on the motherboard for expansion cards. If nothing else it should make sure that they take you more seriously as a purchaser. Thinking about future upgrades now will certainly pay off in the future, whatever you plan to use your PC for.

What happens when something goes wrong?

Unfortunately, when you use a PC, the assumption has to be that something will go wrong at some point! As already mentioned, new versions of *Windows* do come with very sophisticated self-repair facilities, and this should mean that some problems will be fixed without any trouble. However, it is unlikely that this will cover all eventualities. The Internet is now a vast source of information and guidance on computing matters and it is likely that you will be able to find suggestions on how to fix problems such as virus infections, and even software "patches" which will fix problems in the programming that have arisen since the software you are using was written.

Despite this you should still assume that over the lifetime of your PC you will need to seek expert assistance. Potentially the cheapest way to get access to this is through a guarantee provided by the manufacturer or retailer at the point of sale. My experience is that you should try to pay as little for this as you can (I've certainly known a support company go out of business within the life of a contract) and if it is offered for free (or a nominal charge) then it's a good reason for choosing a particular vendor. But do check the small print for exclusions, and remember that a PC is very bulky and heavy – if the service is provided 'on site' or includes free pick-up and delivery then that will make your life much easier and save money too. One of the most important things you can do to 'protect' yourself, is to install anti-virus software and make regular back-ups of your data, both whilst you work and by saving important documents to floppy disk or CD.

Sources of advice and training

Many people start using a PC and manage perfectly well, learning as they go along, without following any formal training programme. However, you may well feel that some instruction would be helpful, and make the whole experience less stressful. In this case there really is a wealth of information and support out there for you to choose from. Despite PCs being a cornerstone of our "digital age", the printed word has much to contribute and it is clear that books on computing continue to be produced in great quantity. There are at least two series which aim to meet the needs of beginners, and increasingly organisations like the Consumers' Association have produced "how to" guides aimed at the non-expert (see the *Further information* section below).

However, if you feel that some hands-on guidance would be more appropriate then there is a wide range of training available usually in small groups. There are a lot of courses provided by commercial training organisations which are very professional, but which are also quite costly. A better bet would be courses provided by a professional body (such as the Royal Society of Medicine's Fellows' IT Training [FiTT] courses), your local library or through the local Education Authority's evening classes which should cover a wide range of PC skills. One recent initiative which should help to increase the range of affordable courses is the European Computer Driving Licence (ECDL) which aims to set a minimum agreed standard of PC skills, which can be tested to a uniform standard in a range of institutions ranging from public libraries to further education colleges. This initiative has been adopted by a number of public bodies including the NHS, and you should be able to find out more from the ECDL website.

This has been a very short overview of how we believe a computer can help you in retirement, but we hope that it has whetted your appetite for more, and perhaps reassured you that in this case it's never too late to learn a new skill and indeed broaden your horizons. Happy computing!

IS

Further information

This is just a small selection of what is available, and if these don't meet your needs there are plenty of alternatives.

Books

Complete Idiot's Guide to the Internet – Peter Kent, and others in this series published by Que, Indianapolis.

The Doctor's Internet Handbook – Robert Kiley, published by RSM Press, London.

A Guide to Healthcare Resources on the Internet – Robert Kiley, ed., published by RSM Press, London.

PCs For Dummies – Dan Gookin, and others in the *For Dummies* series published by Hungry Minds Inc., New York.

The Patient's Internet Handbook – Robert Kiley and Elizabeth Graham, published by RSM Press, London.

The Which? Computer Trouble-shooter – Will Garside, published by Which? Ltd, London.

The Which? Guide to Computers – Richard Wentk, published by Which? Ltd, London.

The Which? Guide to the Internet – Richard Wentk, published by Which? Ltd, London.

Magazines

.net monthly £4.99 with CD; website: www.netmag.co.uk

Internet Magazine monthly £3.75 with CD or book; website: www.internet-magazine.com

PC Advisor monthly £4.99 with DVD; website: www.pcadvisor.co.uk

PC Home monthly £4.99 with CD; website: www.paragon.co.uk/mags/pchome.html

PC Pro monthly £4.99 with DVD; website: www.pcpro.co.uk

He@lth Information on the Internet, RSM Press, London; website: www.rsm.ac.uk/pub/hii.htm

Manufacturers/resellers

Compaq/HP	Telephone: 0845 270 4215, or see website: www.compaq.co.uk/shop/
Dell	Telephone: 0870 907 5818, or see website: www.dell.co.uk
Tiny	Telephone: 0800 783 9812, or see website: www.tiny.com/uk
PC World	Telephone: 0800 056 5732, or see website: www.pcworld.co.uk

Training

- The *Royal Society of Medicine* offers a range of courses suitable for beginners, covering PC use, the Internet, and Microsoft Office. More details can be found on the RSM website, www.rsm.ac.uk
- *European Computer Driving Licence*, the international PC skills standard. Several qualifications can be achieved, see website, www.ecdl.co.uk

(Information correct May 2002)

CHAPTER 13

Entertainment in retirement

One of the joys of retirement is that it allows us to pursue interests which have been denied us during a busy professional life, and it is vitally important that the seemingly long days of retirement should be filled with worthwhile activities. Entertainment of one sort or another will feature largely in most retirements and it is surprising how readily the waking hours can be filled.

Inevitably much of our entertainment will be passive and in most towns there is an embarrassment of riches; for anyone visiting or living in London it is virtually impossible not to find ways of filling the days. Featuring prominently are the arts – theatre, opera and ballet, music, cinema, museums and art galleries, and literature. For much of our entertainment we must go out to public places but there are many opportunities nowadays for entertainment in the home, including television, radio, recordings and reading.

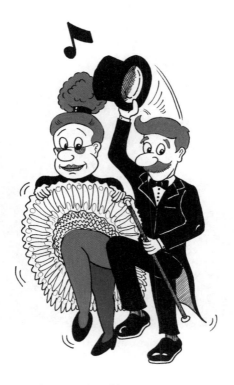

Public entertainment

Theatre

Theatre probably attracts more people to London than any other form of entertainment and for visitors and natives alike, an evening at the theatre – or matinée for those who go to bed early (and have older persons' concessions) – is always an enjoyable experience, provided of course that the play and its actors are good. Apart from dozens of theatres in the West End, there are many other London theatres of equally high quality such as those at Richmond and Wimbledon and the wonderful little Tricycle theatre in Kilburn. Outside London the Royal Shakespeare Company theatre at Stratford-upon-Avon (Figure 1) and the Theatres Royal at Brighton and Windsor are but three examples of numerous venerable theatres which enjoy widespread support.

In addition to "straight" plays many of our theatres promote highly popular musicals such a *Les Misérables, My Fair Lady* and the ubiquitous Lloyd Webber productions. Every year as Christmas approaches, many theatres throughout the United Kingdom turn their attention to their traditional pantomime. With its well-cushioned male dame, its leggy female principal boy and its star comic, pantomime is a singularly British institution which invites more audience participation than any other form of theatre; with the singers and dancers, the pie slingers, the funny hats and masks, and the flashing lights in goggles and wands, pantomime has magic ingredients for children of all ages, including those who have retired, and not just their offspring's offspring.

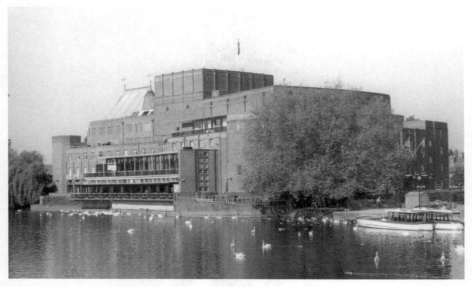

Figure 1   The Royal Shakespeare Company theatre at Stratford-upon-Avon; courtesy of Shakespeare Birthplace Trust, Stratford-Upon-Avon

Opera and ballet

The hapless home of British opera is the Royal Opera House at Covent Garden, London (see Figure 2) and despite a massively expensive refurbishment and repeated panics, it continues to survive. By its very nature opera is, of course, an expensive art form, requiring a conductor, several principal singers, a chorus, an orchestra, and a sizeable backstage staff of dressers, make-up artists, stage managers and lighting operators, to say nothing of box-office staff, programme sellers, bar tenders etc. One might suggest it would be more affordable and accessible to a greater number of people were it not for the monstrous fees paid to maestros, divas and tubby tenors.

London also hosts the English National Opera at the Coliseum and in the summer season, opera is performed at other venues including Holland Park and Kenwood House. Outside London opera is also performed at the renowned Glyndebourne festival in Sussex, at Grange in Hampshire and at Garsington in Oxfordshire, where the intervals between each act can be occupied by champagne picnics on the lawns – weather permitting. However, most major

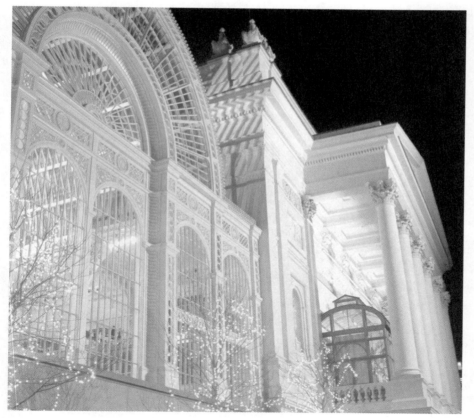

Figure 2   The Royal Opera House, Covent Garden, London; courtesy of R.Moore, 2001

cities provide opera and ballet which are widely publicised in the national and local press, so we need not travel too great a distance for a performance.

In addition to opera, the Royal Opera House also promotes highly successful and popular ballet by such companies as the Royal Ballet, the San Francisco Ballet and the Kirov Ballet. Some excellent ballet can also be seen at Sadler's Wells, and at many other houses outside London.

If you are travelling further afield, many cities throughout the world have famous opera houses: Aix-en-Provence, Milan, Prague, Verona, Zurich, New York, Sydney. If you happen to be in or near Rome during the summer, nocturnal operas are performed in the ancient Baths of Caracalla, beginning late in the evening, at a time when the traffic noise has subsided to a level at which the music becomes audible. Every performance is punctuated by the incessant flashing of cameras, and in every interval the *ragazzi* bound up and down the aisles crying "Gelati! Ice cream! Coca-Cola!" It may not be great opera, but it is great fun. Yet, for sheer spectacle, surely nothing can match a performance of *Aida* amid the hallowed temples of Luxor in Egypt.

Music

To anyone who loves music, residence in or near London is a priceless gift, for London is arguably the musical capital of the world today. With four symphony orchestras and several major concert halls, notably on the South Bank, Kensington and the Barbican Centre, there is hardly a single day in the year when we cannot listen to music of the highest quality. In the summer months

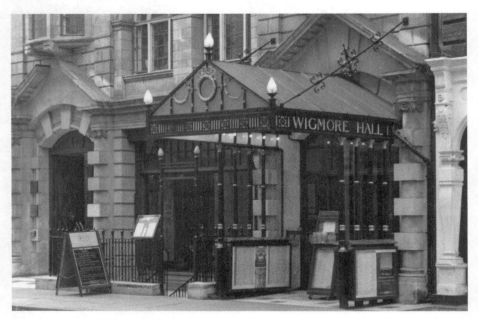

Figure 3 The Wigmore Hall, London

much of it is taken over by the Royal Albert Hall, which houses the world-famous 'Proms' (promenade concerts), jointly founded over 100 years ago by the late Henry Wood with his laryngologist friend George Cathcart.

For smaller musical ensembles, the South Bank also boasts two smaller halls, the Queen Elizabeth Hall and the Purcell Room, while just around the corner from the Royal Society of Medicine is the incomparable Wigmore Hall (see Figure 3), which, with its remarkable acoustic and its inspirational director, William Lyne, attracts international artists of the highest calibre like bees to the honey pot. This amazing hall promotes song recital series, chamber music series, early music and baroque series, pianoforte series, lunchtime concerts, Sunday morning coffee concerts, jazz, and an educational programme, in addition to an international song competition and public auditions for the Young Concert Artists Trust (YCAT). There are many other concert halls, several of them in such churches as St John's, Smith Square and St James's, Piccadilly. Add to these numerous music societies, including the RSM Music Society who produce several excellent concerts each year, and you shall have music wherever you go.

Needless to say, there are many superb concert halls outside London and amongst the most outstanding are the Philharmonic Hall in Liverpool, the Bridgewater Hall in Manchester and the recent Symphony Hall in Birmingham which claims to have the most perfect acoustic of any symphony hall in the British Isles. There are also regular music festivals in Aldeburgh, Bath, Edinburgh, King's Lynn, Windsor and many more besides. Abroad some of the most famous halls include the Concertgebouw in Amsterdam, Carnegie Hall in New York and the Musikverein in Vienna.

Cinema

For many years cinema was by far the most popular form of entertainment outside the home, but that is no longer so, due no doubt to the introduction and almost universal adoption of television. The result is that practically every cinema has now been refashioned into six or more mini-cinemas, each of them frequently half-empty even when highly rated films are being shown. Personally, I find cinema sound unnecessarily and uncomfortably loud, but it still attracts youth who enjoy popcorn and noise, and a small number of elderly persons, usually in pairs or groups, facing an empty afternoon or evening. It is worth seeking out local 'art-house' cinemas such as the Leeds Hyde Park cinema, the Gloucester Guildhall or the Croydon Clocktower. These independent art centres show a refreshing variety of classic, foreign language and non-Hollywood films, often in vintage surroundings with rather more comfortable volume levels.

Museums and art galleries

In addition to the performing arts there is a plethora of visual arts, housed in museums and art galleries throughout the country. Every city has its own special attractions and London alone has numerous museums. In addition to the British Museum, one of the world's truly great such institutions, there is an excellent and diverse group in South Kensington: the Victoria and Albert Museum, the

Science Museum and the Natural History Museum. Mention should also be made of the Imperial War Museum and the National Maritime Museum at Greenwich, where you can also visit the famous Observatory.

Amongst art galleries, special consideration should be given to the National Gallery with its Sainsbury Wing and the neighbouring National Portrait Gallery in Trafalgar Square, the Royal Academy with its Sackler Wing in Piccadilly, the Tate Britain at Millbank, the Tate Modern at Bankside, and the Hayward Gallery on the South Bank.

As we reach retirement and look back on changes that have occurred during our professional lives, many of us develop a growing interest in the history of medicine, and there are in this country many museums given over to that subject. These are described with commendable lucidity in Sue Weir's well-researched *Guide to Medical Museums in Britain*, published by the RSM Press. Nationwide, newspapers give ample notice about local activities, with details about concessions for those who are entitled to them. For anyone visiting or living in London there is a weekly magazine, *Time Out*, which gives copious information about every form of entertainment you could imagine, including some that retired doctors should not be thinking of!

Home entertainment

Television and radio

Television and radio play an increasing part in home entertainment for an ageing population. Although television produces far too much rubbish, especially in the form of domestic or imported 'soaps' and outdated films, the quality of some broadcasts, particularly nature programmes and documentaries, is quite exceptional. There are now many channels to choose from, including digital, satellite and cable. Furthermore, without so much as leaving your seat, you can now turn any programme off – or on – at the press of a button.

Not surprisingly, television is distinctly less popular today than it was a few years ago and a recent survey has shown that once again radio, with no less than ten national stations and innumerable local stations, has become marginally more popular than television. Some radio programmes are now interactive with e-mail and telephone participation.

Video and audio tapes

Many of the best films are quickly made available on video tapes and at surprisingly little cost. We can now purchase a personal copy to play ourselves on our own television set, so that we can watch them in the comfort of our own homes, at an acceptable level of sound and (usually) without interruptions for commercial breaks. Most of these tapes can be hired, from either commercial shops or public libraries, for single or short-term viewing; but others are so special that we may want to keep them permanently for repeated viewing. Several years ago I had the privilege of hearing, live, the brilliant American musician, Wynton

Marsalis, playing with one of his chamber groups at the Lewisham Jazz festival, and I have an audio recording of his (literally) breath-taking performance of trumpet concertos by Haydn, Hummel and Leopold Mozart. Amongst the video tapes that I have recorded for repeated viewing and listening is one such from a programme devised and presented by him in which he expounds on the principles of sonata form to a bunch of bright-eyed kids, spellbound at Tanglewood, summer home of Boston Symphony Orchestra. Pure magic!

We can also listen to music and the spoken word on compact discs (CDs) or magnetic tapes, but several recording companies now record only on CD and it would appear that the days of the tape may be numbered. Most of the books transferred to CDs and tapes are very well produced. These can be bought or rented, and there is a welcome *Talking Books Service*, who supply a wide range of audio materials especially appreciated by people who are unable to read through eyesight problems (details in *Further Information* section).

As an habitual concert-goer I would miss the real "stringiness" of stringed instruments, the occasional tuning of instruments between movements and the general ambience of a live performance if I had to confine my listening to CDs, but what a blessing it is once in a while, to be able to listen to a whole sonata or song cycle or symphony without a single cough!

In recent years there has been a growing interest in the digital versatile disc (DVD) – and it is truly versatile. It does all the things that can be done by videotapes and CDs with superior visual and sound quality. It brings films, documentaries, opera and ballet and music in all its forms to the home – and it brings them in their entirety. Within the next few years it will almost certainly supersede all that has gone before, to become the most popular form of home entertainment within a single package.

Reading

There can be few greater pleasures than reading a good book. One of my own greatest joys in retirement has been to take a holiday thousands of miles away, remote from any telephones or other distractions, for long enough to read one of the truly great modern classics, Vikram Seth's *A Suitable Boy* – the longest novel ever written (so far) in the English language. There is also much to be said for bed-time reading, especially in the subtle form of the short story: one short story, lights out, and off to the Land of Nod.

It is easy enough, if somewhat extravagant, to buy books, but we have many first-class libraries in this country. In my own area we are fortunate to have an outstanding public library which houses, for example, not just a bounteous supply of fiction but also a very comprehensive selection of reference works, including a very active local history section, and a music section which contains an extensive selection of books about music and musicians, scores of much of the classical and modern repertoire, and all 29 volumes of the second (2001) edition of the monumental *New Grove Dictionary of Music and Musicians*.

A great deal of time can be spent reading the daily newspapers which is something we never had time to do as busy doctors. There is also a mind-boggling range of magazines to occupy us, available via subscription or the newsagent. *The Oldie* magazine, for example, carries a wide range of features and reviews aimed at the older audience, but as they say "we do not review stairlifts ... but *The Oldie* will be a splendid read while you are trying to remember where you put your glasses".

The Retired Fellows' Society

A *Retired Fellows' Society* was founded at the Royal Society of Medicine in 1997 (described in detail in chapter 1). It holds four or more intramural events per year in the Society building and several extramural events which have included visits to the National Theatre, guided tours of Soho and the Royal Botanic Gardens and a visit to Portsmouth to see the *Mary Rose*. In addition to topics of medical interest it has also organised meetings of wider appeal for non-medical spouses and other members and guests. These have included talks on *Enigma: Breaking the Code in the Second World War* by Peter Jarvis, *Morse and Me* by Colin Dexter, *Elgar's Malvern* by John Harcup, and *The Arts in Hospitals* by Susan Loppert, Director of Hospital Arts at the Chelsea and Westminster Hospital and a recent winner of the Creative Britons Award.

All the forms of entertainment described here are, of course, passive in nature, and greater satisfaction can be gained by more active forms, such as painting and sculpture, amateur dramatics, choral singing, playing a musical instrument either alone or in groups, or concert management, each involving active participation in areas of personal interest. Chapters on these and other activities are covered elsewhere in this book.

I was delighted to read, in Professor John Stein's article on "Entry requirements for medical school" in *A Career in Medicine: do you have what it takes?* that some medical schools are now encouraging prospective medical students to take at least one arts subject at A-level to complement the compulsory science subjects. In his short story, *At the Pharmacy*, Anton Chekhov wrote: "Science and medicine may change over the years, but the fragrance of a pharmacy is as eternal as the atom". Be that as it may, the pharmacopoeia has escalated out of all recognition since Chekhov's days and these developments in medical science have allowed hundreds of thousands, probably millions of people, to live way beyond Mark Twain's "Scriptural statute of limitations".

Science prolongs active life; the arts make it worthwhile.

JCB

Further information

- Talking Book Service, RNIB Falcon Park, Neasden Lane, London NW10 1TB. Telephone: 020 8438 9000; fax: 020 8438 9001; e-mail: cservices@rnib.org.uk
- *The Oldie Magazine* website: www.theoldie.co.uk; for subscriptions telephone: 020 8545 2757 or fax: 020 8545 2758.

CHAPTER 14

In and out of politics and medicine

"What," you may ask, "has a retired parliamentarian to contribute to a book designed for retiring medical practitioners?" There is an immediate answer: the contrast in one's circumstances and status. The planned retirement of a doctor from a lifelong professional practice is rather different from the not infrequent, sudden and often unexpected departure from parliamentary politics. However unexpected retirement is, of course, sometimes forced upon doctors for a variety of reasons. My thoughts may offer some insight into the special needs and personal problems that confront someone who is unprepared for the end of their employed life. It may give some suggestions in recognising, responding to and treating withdrawal symptoms. My contribution will be, something of a personal odyssey, anecdotal and autobiographical in approach.

Why not get involved politics?

Politics these days is regarded as a young man's profession – I say man's because sadly there are still too few women. Ambitious young men, aspiring to a seat at the Cabinet table will commence their career with involvement in student politics at university. On graduating, they seek employment in a politics-related occupation: research assistant to an MP or desk officer in a party HQ while simultaneously seeking election to a local authority. This has become the career apprenticeship for prospective parlimentary candidates of the main political parties. To some extent it is a good thing – politics needs youth, energy, enthusiasm and new ideas but these politicians come from an enclosed political world. There is, however, a real need to redress this imbalance – to have a leavening of maturity, experience and understanding of the ways of the world beyond the political hothouse. Herein lies the opportunity and challenge to those who have these characteristics. Medical practitioners are well-qualified, perhaps uniquely qualified, to bring their skills of analysis and diagnosis, judgement and decision and fresh ideas to the political process, especially in the all-important and politically sensitive field of healthcare.

With the increase in the number of health trusts, charity trusteeships, boards of school governors, consultative groups, local authorities and many other areas where political decisions are made, there is a need for experienced and socially-aware men and women. It is in these areas that a retired medical practitioner can play a positive role. Some of these appointments are on a voluntary basis, whilst some carry a small honorarium or pay a little more. Appointments to such boards or candidatures are often through nomination or recommendation of the local party political organisation. So it is necessary to offer one's services through the party political route. Those who have no wish necessarily to define themselves with a political party but would like to serve in some way could write to The Public Appointments Unit, who maintain a register of those who express interest (see *Further information* section for contact details).

Of course, having been in politics myself, I would suggest you can go for gold, give it your best shot and stand directly for parliament at a general election on a simple issue of local concern. It has been done before and the retired consultant, Dr Richard Taylor, did it successfully at the last election in June 2001. He headed the *Health Concern* campaign to stop Kidderminster hospital being downgraded, and stood as an independent candidate, taking the Wyre Forest seat in Kidderminster with a majority of 17,630 votes.

It is equally important to remember that there is an increasing percentage of older people in our communities today and consequently an increasing need for them to be involved in political debate. They need to contribute their skills and experience to politics and be properly represented, rather than opting out. Len Overy-Owen, as another example, set up the Grey Party in 2000 to campaign in Colchester for pensioners' rights and concerns. Good luck to them both and good luck to you.

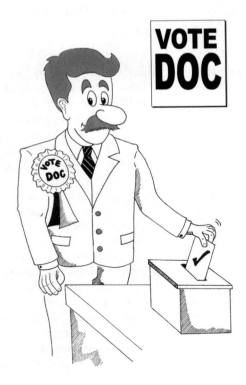

Retirement for a politician

"Retirement" is hardly the right word for this parliamentarian's rite of passage. Most political careers, however, as it has been so often noted, end in either defeat, disgrace, or, at the very least, in disappointment and tears. Rarely can a departure from parliament be planned. This is the dilemma, it is predictable, you can see it coming but you cannot properly prepare for it with a well-researched retirement strategy. Any sitting MP approaching a general election must do it in the confidence he will win, however unpromising the prospects and predictions. He must persuade himself that he will win and communicate this confidence to his supporters and helpers. Any wavering from this confidence and he will feel and look like a loser. Enquiries about alternative employment or talk of the garden and the grandchildren is detrimental to the psychological focus on winning the election.

Since there is no fixed retirement age for Members of Parliament, there is no imperative for members sitting in safe seats to retire. They often stay on beyond what would be the customary retirement age of 65. Unlike medicine there is always a good reason to stay on for "Just one more Parliament – good to have some experienced old hands on the back benches to help the Government (or Opposition) through the testing time ahead – give the constituency sufficient time to choose a suitable successor."

The tea room of the House of Commons is the nerve centre of rumour and gossip. At breakfast time one Monday morning I met a colleague, an elderly and long-standing member, in pensive mood. He mentioned with a contrived casual remark that he was "thinking of standing down at the next election". My colleague's professional background was at the bar, though it was many years since he last held a brief. He mused about the future. "In the old days when I first came into this House you could expect to retire with the offer of a County Court judgeship, or at least a Governorship of some small dependency you had probably never heard of. Now you must think yourself lucky if you are offered a seat on the Milk Marketing Board."

Few such jobs are available to doctors who retire early through ill-health or some misdemeanour. While some politicians can retire from politics to take up more prestigious or well-paid work in places like the European Commission or the banking sector, few in the medical profession possess the appropriate business skills and experience to make such a career move.

Initial feelings of loss

The challenges to a politician retiring are manifold and perhaps the greatest is the enveloping sense of rejection and loss of a whole way of life. A politician's routine requires his presence at Westminster for part of the week, and for the remainder in his constituency where often the family home is situated, with wife and children very much in the public eye. Medicine dictates one's way of life and involvement with patients and their problems in much the same way as constituency duties – rewarding and absorbing at the time and inevitably much missed upon retirement.

Members of Parliament and doctors alike are never really off duty until retirement when everything suddenly stops – in my case when still young and active. I had a sense of loss, like a bereavement, bringing with it a grieving and mourning process. There is a perceptible loss of self-confidence, and to some degree a loss of identity accompanied by a more material loss of income. But people can be kind as they are to the bereaved; they send supportive letters with advice, "You will be able to spend more time with the family; catch up with your friends and have more leisure activities", and some invite you to a nice lunch.

Devising a strategy to cope

How did I cope with this loss on a personal and a professional level? A wise friend who was with me during the hours awaiting poll results at my first election suggested I should write on one side of a postcard all the things I would like to do (but would not be able to do) if I were elected. They were not particularly outrageous things but simple pleasures, like theatre, books and country weekends. I kept this card as a talisman, and referred to it when I did in fact lose my seat. I would recommend this sort of exercise to anyone who is facing retirement – it focuses one's mind positively and constructively on the future.

I was 57 when I retired from parliament, defeated at the General Election. It seemed too early for an enforced early retirement, I needed a purposeful occupation and I needed an income. Parliamentary or NHS pensions require long-service to be adequate and mine was relatively short. I was, therefore, looking for a job and without delay, and I did not expect a call from the Milk Marketing Board! I put myself about in the wider world of business and commerce. Potential employers, ever courteous, clearly had reservations.

I reviewed my position. I was a widower with all my children financially independent so only really had to consider myself. I developed my personal retirement plan, identifying my aims, prioritising my objectives and using my strengths in order to generate sufficient income to live in a modest but comfortable style. I wanted a paid occupation that was not only congenial, but positively enjoyable. I wanted a varied working life, time to pursue both old and new interests, and broad social activity.

I devised a CV (which my children said read more like a rake's progress than a planned career path). I had done a number of very different jobs which I would explain by saying that I recognised the importance of gaining "transferable skills" early in life in different work areas. In seeking variety in work why not seek two part-time jobs rather than one full-time job? I was seeking a "portfolio career" before management-speak had identified and labelled it thus. I read law at university and although had been called to the bar, I had never seriously practised. I had worked in the advertising and marketing industry, before moving to a property investment company, where the law of planning and landlord and tenant were called into play. While with this company, in the interest of my health and safety at work, I had qualified as a chartered surveyor. Before entering parliament I had also held an academic post teaching property law. The aspect of this varied career path which I had found the most rewarding was teaching so I sought my future in my pre-parliamentary past.

Clearly, most doctors haven't had such a varied career path upon which to draw but there are many strands of a doctor's experience that may suggest a fulfilling occupation for one's time after retirement. Many of these options are described elsewhere in this book. However, one can and should approach such a situation in a positive way, cast aside negative feelings and resist passive acceptance.

GB

Further information

- The Public Appointments Unit, Room 030, 70 Whitehall, London SW1A 2PS, or see www.cabinet-office.gov.uk/quango/index/pubapp.htm on the internet

CHAPTER 15

Pensions, inheritance and tax planning

Pensions

The subject of pension provision for the medical profession is complex. This short chapter outlines the provisions made by the government and details how additional provisions for retirement can be made. (You may find more information about government pensions in *CAB and Benefits*, p 93.) Before considering pensions, those with dependants, spouses or partners, and minor children for example, should consider whether they have sufficient protection against "catastrophe" risks.

It is all very well attempting to maximise income in retirement but a greater priority should be:

1. Adequate life assurance on both spouses or partners
2. Critical illness insurance to enable capital liabilities, such as a mortgage, to be discharged in the event a heart attack, a stroke, kidney failure, etc. (The details of the illnesses covered are listed in the policy document.)
3. Income protection insurance (also known as permanent health insurance) to provide a long term income in the event of disability

In simple terms, members of the profession in the United Kingdom qualify for membership of the National Health Service Pension Scheme (NHSPS). Membership applies to:

- General practitioners (GPs) who are self-employed and taxed under Schedule D
- Hospital doctors and consultants who are employees and taxed under Schedule E.

Members of each category contribute 6% of pensionable pay whilst the NHS pays 7% of pensionable pay. Contributions normally cease at age 65. A GP's pensionable pay is defined as gross NHS fees reduced by an agreed "expenses" percentage. For employees pensionable pay is defined as annual pay plus certain regular allowances but excluding overtime and travelling expenses.

For GPs who generally retire between the ages of 60 and 70, the pension is 1.4% of the career pensionable pay uprated to the date of retirement in line with pay levels which are in force at the time that the individual stops paying contributions. Pensionable service may not exceed 45 years. For employees, the pension is 1/80th of final year's pensionable pay for each year of the scheme membership – this is limited to 40 years at the age of 60. In addition, at retirement members receive a lump sum of three times the pension which is tax free.

If the member dies in service, there is a lump sum payment for employees of twice pensionable pay whilst for GPs the lump sum is twice the average uprated pensionable pay. In addition, if membership has been at least two years at the date of death, a spouse's pension is payable which will depend on the member's age and length of service. A child allowance may also be paid.

Members who will not be able to achieve maximum service by the time they retire may be able to buy additional years service to enable them to increase their benefits. These additional benefits can be purchased by a single payment within 12 months of joining the scheme, or within 12 months of marriage, or by the member paying increased contributions on a regular basis.

There are various ways in which members of the profession can top up their NHSPS benefits:

(a) Doctors taxed under Schedule E

- They can pay additional voluntary contributions (AVCs) or free standing AVCs (FSAVCs) of up to 9% of pensionable pay on top of their normal member's contribution of 6% (the maximum contribution by a member is 15% of earnings)

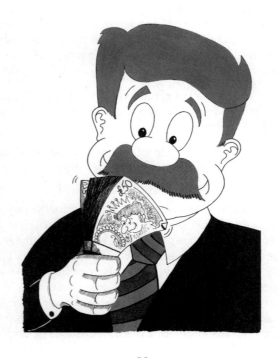

- They can pay contributions to a stakeholder or personal pension plan, the amount of the premium being calculated by reference to earnings from private practice. The percentage is governed by the age at the start of the fiscal year and the earnings limited to a figure (the earnings cap) laid down by the Chancellor (£97,200 for 2002–2003).
- They may be able to pay £3,600 gross to a stakeholder or personal pension if their earnings do not exceed £30,000 per annum. This limit may change in the future. Such payments are made net of basic rate tax and potentially qualify for higher rate tax relief.

(b) Doctors taxed under Schedule D

- GPs can forego their tax relief on NHS contributions and contribute to a stakeholder or personal pension in respect of both NHS pensionable and private earnings up to the earnings cap.

As will be apparent, this subject is complicated and this article merely scratches the surface. The value of professional advice cannot be over-estimated, particularly in the area of additional protection against catastrophic risks.

DB

Wills and inheritance

It is an often quoted fact that two things in life are inevitable: death and taxes, and, as if this is not bad enough, in many cases death can be the cause of taxes! However, with some forethought and planning, not only can you make life a little easier for those you leave behind but also alleviate the impact of tax on your estate after death.

Why bother to make a will?

For many reasons. Setting out exactly how you wish your estate to pass on your death, appointing executors and trustees to deal with your assets, setting out clear funeral wishes and, if appropriate, appointing guardians for any minor children are all excellent reasons for making a will.

Appointing executors

Executors are those chosen by the testator to administer his or her estate. An executor's authority starts from the moment of death. It is usually confirmed by a court order known as the Grant of Probate. In an intestate estate, i.e. where there is no will or the will in whole or part is not valid, an administrator is appointed to act and his authority stems only from the date of the appointment. This means that where there is no will or no valid appointment of an executor in a will, there will be a hiatus pending the court order where nobody has authority to deal with the estate.

Guardians

The appointment of guardians of minor children either to act with the surviving spouse, or in the case of the second spouse to die, is obviously important. This is especially relevant in cases where the surviving partner does not have parental responsibility for the child, e.g. in cases of non marriage or second marriages.

Intestacy

A full or partial intestacy can occur where there is either no will at all or the will fails to deal with either the appointment of executors or the distribution of all or part of the estate. The rules of intestacy, as far as the distribution of estates is concerned, mean that husbands and wives do not automatically inherit from each other. In fact, these rules are quite complex, depending on the size of the estate and the composition of the deceased's family. A summary of these rules is as follows:

Where there is a surviving spouse

- If there are children or grandchildren, the surviving spouse will take all personal chattels, a fixed sum of £125,000 and a life interest (i.e. the right to the income but not the capital) in half the remainder of the estate. The other half will pass to the children (or grandchildren if children have pre-deceased) and will be held on trust if any of these are under 18.
- If there are no children/grandchildren but there is a surviving parent or, if no parent, a surviving brother or sister, the surviving spouse, once again, will receive all the personal chattels. They will also receive a fixed sum of £200,000 and half of the balance of the estate outright. The remaining half will pass to the parent or, if no parent, to the deceased's siblings in equal shares or to their children if they have predeceased.
- If there are no other relatives, the surviving spouse will inherit the entire estate.

Where there is no surviving spouse

- If there are children, then the entire estate will pass to them or to their children if they have predeceased.
- If there are no children, the estate will pass to the following family members in order so that no person receives any part of the estate if there is someone in a higher category:
  - Parents (in equal shares, if appropriate).
  - Brothers and sisters of the whole blood or their issue if any of them have predeceased leaving children. The share of any beneficiary under the age of 18 to be held on trust.
  - Brothers and sisters of the half blood and their issue as above.
  - Grandparents (if more than one in equal shares).
  - Uncles and aunts of the whole blood or their children if they have predeceased (once again, held upon trust for any beneficiary under 18).

- Uncles and aunts of the half blood or their issue as above.
- The Crown/Duchy of Lancaster/Duke of Cornwall.

This means that, in some cases, the deceased's estate could be distributed to quite distant relatives or, indeed, to the Crown.

The rules also cover the right of the surviving spouse to "capitalise" his or her life interest and to receive a share of the matrimonial home instead of a cash sum.

The above is just a very brief summary of the complex rules of intestacy. How much better, therefore, to avoid these potential difficulties and leave a will dealing with the distribution of the estate, rather than rely upon the statutory rules of intestacy, especially in parts of the country where house prices are so high that the surviving spouse could be left in the unsatisfactory position of not owning outright the family home.

Tax planning

Inheritance tax is a tax on certain lifetime gifts and, in some circumstances, on death. In the moment before death, each and every person is deemed to make a "transfer" of their estate, which is potentially taxable at 40 per cent above the threshold set by the government. This threshold, known as the "nil-rate band", is currently £250,000 and this usually has an inflationary increase in the Chancellor's budget every year.

"Transfers", i.e. lifetime gifts and assets passing on death between UK domiciled spouses, are exempt from inheritance tax and so are gifts to charity. Certain business assets and interests in a business and agricultural property are also exempt from inheritance tax. Assuming the value of your estate to be large enough, it is possible to save £96,800 of inheritance tax by passing the "nil-rate band" straight to the next generation either by outright gift or on trust, although care must be taken to ensure that the surviving spouse is adequately provided for.

If you require a more complex type of will involving inheritance tax planning, or advice on lifetime tax planning then it is essential to consult a solicitor specialising in this area.

HF

RSM Press is also grateful for the advice of Tony Charles from the Medical Sickness Society on this chapter.

CHAPTER 16

Citizens' Advice Bureaux and old age benefits – your rights

Why do over 5 million people go to the Citizens' Advice Bureaux each year?

Life has become more demanding than ever for many people and particularly as they get older. This is mirrored in the growing amount of work which Citizens' Advice Bureaux (CAB) are tackling every day. The CAB service is the largest advice service in the country with more than 2,000 outlets. It is free, independent, confidential and impartial. CAB pride themselves on providing a service for everyone which is delivered professionally by fully trained voluntary and paid staff. Ninety per cent of people who work in CAB are volunteers.

For over 60 years the CAB service has been serving local communities. Each CAB is locally run and the advisers have access to a national information system which is centrally prepared and updated each month. As well as giving information and advice, practical help can be given with filling out forms, drafting letters and negotiating on the client's behalf with other agencies such as government departments and local tax and benefits offices. Bureaux have to ensure that they are accessible for people with mobility problems and hearing impairment, and many are able to deliver specialist telephone and home visiting services for older people and disabled people.

Information and advice are crucial elements in enabling people to take control of their lives. Without help many people find it impossible to cope with the complexity of today's world. It is a paradox that the people who are most overwhelmed with bureaucracy – forms, means tests, reviews, demands for information – are benefit claimants, a large proportion of whom are the long-term sick, disabled and older people. Without someone to help them exercise their rights and responsibilities, people can easily be marginalised. This is especially true for those who are frail, disabled or retired.

The CAB service also recognises that the long-term solutions for many clients' problems often require changes in the policies and services which are failing to meet their needs. Policy makers and government departments take the views of the CAB seriously because they come directly from the grassroots. The National Association of CAB produces many reports each year based on the first hand experience of their clients.

Bureaux belong to the National Association of Citizens' Advice Bureaux (NACAB), which sets standards for advice, training, equal opportunities and accessibility, co-ordinates national social policy, media, publicity and parliamentary work and produces the national information system in paper and electronic versions. NACAB and each CAB are registered individual charities. CAB receive basic core funding from their local authorities and fundraise to provide other services to meet the needs of the communities they serve whereas NACAB receives its grant from central government to enable it to provide the services mentioned above and run seven regional offices.

The aims of the CAB service are:

- To ensure that individuals do not suffer through lack of knowledge of their rights and responsibilities or of the services available to them, or through an inability to express their needs effectively

And equally:

- To exercise a responsible influence on the development of social policies and services, both locally and nationally.

The CAB service is independent and provides free, confidential and impartial advice to everybody regardless of race, sex, disability, sexuality or class.

The information in this section relating to pensions and benefits for older people is a brief outline of the main conditions and criteria for claimants. It is not possible, within the space available, to go into great detail. Benefit and pension rates change annually and I have deliberately not quoted amounts which can be claimed. Government departments may also change their name. For example, the Department of Social Security has now become the Department for Work and Pensions.

The rules which apply to all benefits are strict and often complicated. It is therefore advisable to seek the help of a CAB adviser or specialist Welfare Benefits adviser in order to ensure you are claiming the right benefit and that you meet all the criteria. The forms themselves can appear daunting at first. Advisers are experienced in helping people to complete them. In our experience claim forms completed correctly are more likely to be successful.

Retirement pensions

There are three main categories of retirement pension.

- Category A – payable on your own National Insurance contribution record.
- Category B – payable by virtue of your spouse's NI record and only available to married women, widows or widowers. There are different conditions for claiming depending on whether you are a married woman, widow or widower.
- Category D – payable to those over 80 years old and this is non-contributory, (i.e. not dependent on your National Insurance contribution record).

The vast majority of men receive Category A retirement pension. Women usually receive either Category A or Category B retirement pensions, but may sometimes be able to claim both.

When you reach "pensionable age" which is currently 65 for a man and 60 for a woman, you become entitled to retirement pension. The pensionable age for women will be increased from 60 to 65 between 2010 and 2020. All women born after 5 April 1955 will reach pensionable age at 65.

You must claim your retirement pension. You are not automatically entitled to it just because you reach pensionable age. If you do not claim you will be treated as having deferred your retirement. It is not compulsory to retire and you can choose whether or not to give up work. Similarly, you might want to retire before pensionable age. You will not receive any state retirement pension until you reach your pensionable age, but you should ensure that you are protecting your national insurance record. Special rules apply to divorcees, widows and widowers.

If you have not spent all your working life in the UK your pension may be affected. There may, however, be reciprocal arrangements with the country/countries in which you have worked which may help you. If you have worked in another European Economic Area (EEA) state you may benefit from European Community (EC) law. Your pension will not be uprated should you go abroad once you have retired, unless you are going to another EEA state or to a country with whom the UK has reciprocal arrangements.

You may want to defer your retirement and your entitlement to your retirement pension. You can do this for a period of up to five years after reaching pensionable age. However, if you are a married man, entitled to a Category A pension and your wife is entitled to a Category B pension by virtue of your contributions, you cannot defer your retirement without your wife's consent; unless it is unreasonably withheld. You must notify the Pension Service, which is part of the Department for Work and Pensions of your intention to defer your retirement. This is known as "de-retiring". You can do this at any time during the first five years after reaching pensionable age. You can cancel your deferment at anytime but you cannot then de-retire a second time.

It is, however, important to consider the following if you are thinking of deferring your retirement. If you defer entitlement to your pension for the whole five year period you will receive about 37 per cent extra retirement pension each week. However, you may be better off claiming it and investing it because if you die within five years of reaching pensionable age any money invested will go to your family, but if you die before you claim, only your spouse will benefit from the deferment of your pension.

Retirement pensions are taxable, except for increases for children (i.e. you may have children under 16 and/or 19 years old). It is possible to receive retirement pension and some income support and thus other means-tested benefits such as housing benefit and/or council tax benefit. Pensioners receive a higher rate of some means-tested benefits. However, their retirement pensions are taken fully into account in the calculations. Being in receipt of retirement pension provides a passport to other benefits, for example, people over 60 get free prescriptions and eye tests regardless of income.

In England, Wales and Scotland you can contact the National Tele-Claim Service to request a claim form or provide details over the phone in order to make your claim. The number is:

0845 300 1084 (textphone 0845 300 2086) 0700h to 1900h Mon–Fri.

Graduated Retirement Benefit

This benefit can still be paid to a person over retirement age even if they do not meet the requirements to receive a retirement pension because they do not satisfy the national insurance contribution conditions. Between 1961 and 6 April 1975 people who paid flat rate Class 1 contributions also paid graduated contributions. For every £7.50 contributed by a man and £9 by a woman during that period, they are now entitled to £9.06 per week. The contribution conditions for graduated retirement benefit discriminate against women on the grounds of their sex, but are probably not contrary to EC law.

State Earnings Related Pension Scheme (SERPS)

This scheme is for those who have paid Class 1 national insurance contributions in excess of the minimum required in order to receive retirement and widows pensions. SERPS is to be replaced by a new scheme in April 2002 and will target those on low and moderate incomes. The regulations and conditions with regard to SERPS are complex and you should seek advice from your local CAB, the Pension Service or a pensions adviser. Different rules apply depending on whether you reached pensionable age before 6 April 1999 or after 5 April 1999.

If you are widowed on or after 6 October 2002 you may not be able to receive 100 per cent of the SERPS based on your deceased spouse's contributions. The percentage of SERPS you can inherit depends on when your spouse reaches pension age. There has already been some advance publicity about this in order to allow people to make alternative arrangements if they wish to do so.

Pensions Forecasts

You can find out how much pension you are likely to get by completing form BR19 available from your local social security office. The forecast includes how much basic, additional and graduated pension you will get and how many extra contributions are needed to qualify for a minimum or full pension. The form should be sent to:

Retirement Pension Forecast, RPSA Unit, Pensions and Overseas Benefit Directorate, Newcastle upon Tyne, NE98 1BA; Telephone: 0191 218 7585; for people with hearing difficulties: 0191 218 2160

Bereavement Benefits

If your spouse dies you may qualify for bereavement benefits. There are three main benefits and these are:

- A lump sum payment of £2,000 – Bereavement Payment

- A weekly benefit for widows and widowers who have children – Widowed Parents Allowance. There is no lower age limit, but claimant must be old enough to be legally married.
- A weekly benefit paid for 52 weeks to widows or widowers who are at least 45 and under pensionable age when their spouse dies and satisfy national insurance contribution conditions.

You are entitled to bereavement benefits regardless of your level of income and savings. You must claim within three months of your spouse's death. It is very important to claim promptly as payment can only be backdated for three months from when you make your claim.

Attendance Allowance (AA)

If you are over 65 and have care or supervision needs you may qualify for Attendance Allowance. There are two rates, higher and lower for which you must meet certain "disability" conditions. You must have:

- either daytime or night time attention or supervision needs for the lower rate, and
- both daytime and night time requirements or be terminally ill for the higher rate.

You must also have met the conditions for a continuous period of six months. If you are terminally ill you are automatically treated as satisfying the conditions for the higher rate and do not have to wait for six months before qualifying for AA. The "special rules" apply in these cases and your claim for Attendance Allowance should be dealt with within 15 days.

An award for Attendance Allowance can be for either a fixed or indefinite period. It will depend on how long the decision maker estimates your current needs may last. If your award is for a limited period you will need to renew your claim. This can be done from six months before the award runs out. You must report any change in your condition which could alter the amount of your benefit. You could be overpaid benefit which would have to be repaid. Attendance Allowance is not taxable.

You should also contact your local authority to see if you qualify for the Blue Badge Scheme (previously Orange Badge Scheme) of parking concessions which operates throughout Great Britain. There may be certain local variations.

You may also be able to get a grant for home insulation and other heating improvements if a member of your household receives Attendance Allowance or Disability Living Allowance, from the Home Energy Efficiency Scheme. Contact the freephone number for the country in which you live:

England: 0800 952 0600; textphone: 0800 072 0156
Scotland: 0800 072 0150; textphone: 0800 072 0156
Wales: 0800 316 2815; textphone: 0800 072 0156
Northern Ireland: 0800 181 667; textphone: 0191 233 1054
Website: www.eaga.co.uk

Invalid Care Allowance (ICA)

If you are receiving Attendance Allowance and someone regularly looks after you they may be entitled to Invalid Care Allowance. Your carer qualifies for ICA if they care for you at least 35 hours per week, they are not gainfully employed or in full-time education and are aged over 16 and under 65 years old. A claim can be backdated for up to three months. ICA is taxable. The carer is allowed to have temporary breaks from caring for you without losing any benefit. Effectively they can have four weeks holiday within any period of six months. If AA stops because you are in hospital or other special accommodation the ICA also stops.

ICA is regarded as income when calculating means-tested benefits. It is an earnings replacement benefit and people cannot usually receive more than one earnings replacement benefit at a time. It is very important to report any changes in circumstances which could affect your right to ICA. You may have to repay any overpaid benefit if you do not do this.

At present, if the person receiving AA dies, the ICA paid to the carer ceases immediately. The Government is, however, planning to change the rules to enable ICA to continue for eight weeks after the death of the person receiving care.

If you are receiving ICA when you reach 65 you are still treated as though you are receiving ICA even though the retirement pension is higher. However, there are extra rules to retain the carer's premium. Do seek advice at this stage if it applies to you.

There are residence tests which may affect your qualification for AA and ICA. You must:

- Be ordinarily resident in Great Britain *and*
- Be present in Great Britain *and*
- Have been present in Great Britain for 26 weeks during the previous 12 months.

If you are terminally ill you are exempted from the above rule.

Health benefits

Although the National Health Service (NHS), in general, provides free health care, there are some services for which a charge is made.

If you are receiving Income Support and/or you are a permanent resident in a residential care or nursing home (where your place is partly or wholly funded by the local authority) you will be exempt from these charges. You may also qualify for exemption or help with health charges under the low income scheme or on other grounds.

You qualify for free prescriptions and free eye tests once you reach the age of 60. You may also be entitled to help with dental treatment and dentures, wigs and fabric supports, and fares to hospital if your income is low enough, you or a member of your family is receiving Income Support, Working Families Tax Credit, Disabled Person's Tax Credit, or you are a permanent resident in a residential care or nursing home.

Healthcare equipment can be provided by local authorities, hospitals and GPs, either free or on prescription. Some local Red Cross branches may also be able to offer some equipment. Social Services departments can arrange for special equipment but it may be subject to a charge. There are many firms who advertise in national and local newspapers and on TV who provide special equipment and adaptations for older people and the disabled. Some even have showrooms and shops in various towns and cities where you can try out their products.

Housing grants

Your local authority may be able to help with a grant towards the cost of improving your home. The main grants available are:

- Renovation grants
- Disabled facilities grants
- Home repair assistance

Home Energy Efficiency Scheme (HEES) for insulation and draught proofing:

Energy Action Grants Agency, PO Box 1NG, Newcastle upon Tyne, NE99 2RP; freephone: 0800 072 0150; see the websites: www.saveenergy.co.uk and www.eaga.co.uk, for a searchable database of energy-saving grants.

Local authority social services departments have a statutory duty to provide a range of practical and financial help to older people. A variety of help is available for people with an illness or disability to assist with things such as paying for care services in your own home, equipment, transport and holidays.

Getting paid

Once you have made your claim for retirement pension or other benefits you can choose how it is paid. This can be by girocheque, order book or payment direct into your bank or other account four weekly or quarterly in arrears.

Payment of benefit while abroad

Unless there are reciprocal arrangements with other countries or you can rely on EC law it is not normally possible to have British benefits paid to you while you are abroad. However, there are circumstances where it is possible and these are for bereavement benefits, retirement pensions, attendance allowance and invalid care allowance. However, do seek advice to ensure your circumstances meet the criteria laid down for payment of benefits and pension while you are abroad.

If you are living abroad temporarily and can show that you are normally resident in the UK you may still get annual increases in your pension. The increased rate will usually be paid in arrears when you return to the UK. If you are living abroad permanently, you will not normally receive annual increases to your pension unless you are visiting the UK and your visit coincides with a retirement pension payday. However, if you move to another EEA state you can have your retirement pension paid there and it will be uprated each year as it is in the UK.

The Pension Service will advise on the transfer of pensions overseas, medical cover and claiming benefits abroad:

Pensions and Overseas Benefits Directorate, Newcastle upon Tyne, NE98 1BA; overseas customer service line: 0191 218 7878;

website: www.thepensionservice.gov.uk

Going into hospital

The amount of benefit to which you are entitled may be reduced if you go into hospital and remain for a specific length of time. The care component of AA stops after four weeks as an inpatient. ICA stops when the person being cared for loses their AA.

The weekly rate of retirement pension will be reduced after you have been an inpatient for six weeks.

Challenging decisions

You can apply for a revision or supersession of bereavement benefit, retirement pension, attendance allowance and invalid care allowance or appeal against the decision. If you need to do this, I would strongly advise you seek the help of a specialist Welfare Benefits adviser at your local CAB who will help you through the process.

Winter fuel payment

This is an annual tax-free payment made to people who are aged 60 or over. It is not a loan. If you are in receipt of retirement pension the winter fuel payment will be paid automatically.

Winter Fuel Payments Helpline: 0845 915 1515; textphone: 0845 601 5613

Minimum income guarantee

If your income is below a certain amount you may be able to claim minimum income guarantee.

Claimline: 0800 028 11 11 open weekdays between 0700h –1900h; textphone: 0800 028 35 93

Budgeting loans, crisis loans (interest free) and Community Care grants

More information on these and whether you qualify can be obtained from your local social security office. The local office can be found in the phone book or on the Department for Work and Pensions' website: www.dwp.gov.uk.

Driving licences

If you are aged 70 or over, the fee for a three-year driving licence has been cut to £6. You do need to renew it every three years. The Driver and Vehicle Licence

Agency will send you a renewal form just before your 70th birthday. For more information telephone the DVLA: 0870 240 00 09.

Free TV licences

If you are 75 or over, you can now watch many of your favourite programmes for free.
   TV Licensing information line: 0845 602 33 34; BBC website: www.bbc.co.uk

Free admission to national museums and galleries

You may be able to benefit from this if you are aged 60 or over.
   Department of Culture, Media and Sport enquiry line: 020 7211 6200; Website: www.culture.gov.uk/heritage/index.html

Christmas bonus

People who receive retirement pension, attendance allowance and invalid care allowance will qualify for a Christmas bonus of £10. You can claim an extra £10 for your husband or wife (or someone you live with as husband or wife) if you are both over pensionable age. The Christmas bonus is paid automatically, but if you have not received it you must claim within a year, otherwise your right to it is lost. The bonus is not taxable and has no affect on other benefits.

Charities

There are hundreds of charities that provide a variety of help to people in need. Your local authority social services department may know of appropriate charities that could help you, or you can consult publications such as the Guide to Grants for Individuals in Need and the Charities Digest in your local library.

Further information

- As well as Citizens' Advice Bureaux, law centres and local authority welfare rights workers can help with advice and information. The Legal Services Commission have lists of organisations who provide advice in different areas of law as well as welfare benefits. Telephone: 0845 608 1122
- Visit the website: www.justask.org.uk, to search a directory for advisers from the Community Law Service within your area.
- The Department for Work and Pensions, publishes many useful leaflets, which are free from your local office, or telephone: 0800 666 555. Address and phone numbers for your local office are in your local phone book, or check on the websites: www.dss.gov.uk or www.dwp.gov.uk
- Pensions Info-line: 0845 731 3233

- *SeniorLine* is a free Help the Aged phoneline providing information on help and benefits available to people over state pension age and their carers. Telephone: 0808 800 6565 or visit the website: www.helptheaged.org.uk
- For information on a whole range of help and advice available through central and local government see the *Pensioners' Guide* booklet – to get a free copy visit the website: www.info4pensioners.gov.uk or telephone: 0845 6065 065 (7 am–11 pm); textphone: 0845 6064 064.
- Other useful websites:
  The National Association of Citizens' Advice Bureaux: www.nacab.org.uk
  24-hour advice online provided by the CAB: www.adviceguide.org.uk
  For advice about rights and welfare: www.rights.org.uk
  For information about all UK legislation such as Acts of Parliament: www.hmso.gov.uk

I hope this chapter has given you some idea of the rights and benefits available for older people, especially in retirement. The websites and contact telephone numbers are very useful and will provide more detail. (Information correct at May 2002.)

PS

CHAPTER 17

Frailty

In a society which no longer venerates old age and where longevity is viewed for its negative attributes, older people must prepare themselves to be self-reliant in the event of frailty. The demise of the extended family, hastened by the expectation of home ownership, is widely accepted – family members are obliged to work to pay their mortgages on small houses which have no spare space for parents. The nuclear family has no-one at home to care for frail relatives and meagre financial resources to pay for care when it is needed. The state accepted responsibility in 1948 for the vulnerable in society but can no longer raise the taxes necessary to meet the cost. Where does this leave the frailer members of our society? Is an inability to look after them a feature of a civilised society that has lost its way? Perhaps we need the wisdom of old age to help resolve this conundrum!

Planning for possible frailty in older age is best done over a large drink as it requires courage to face one's mortality and to contemplate how best to make adequate provision before physical frailty, dementia, incontinence and whole systems shut down overtakes the decision. There is a bewildering range of choices, many of which require considerable financial investment and, if left until the future is obvious, could already be too late. Frailty occurs at a time when individuals are least well equipped to tackle the confusing maze of options and bureaucracy. It may be especially difficult to settle to this subject as there is possibly an inner voice saying, "it won't happen to me". There is no way of knowing whether you could be one of the 7% of over 65s who require nursing home care.

It will be of little consolation to know that in England by the year 2020 it is forecast that there will be more people retired than working. This consequence of the triumphs of medicine and absence of world wars is causing an ever increasing demand for care in old age. In the face of an ageing population, what are the options available to the 4th Age? At the beginning of the 21st century, can the frail and vulnerable expect the state to make sufficient provision from the cradle to the grave, as envisaged at the inception of the National Health Service? The reality is that the state cannot afford to provide many of these services free of charge. Social policy, irrespective of political persuasion at the beginning of the 21st century, is being planned on the basis of joint or shared responsibility for meeting the cost of care.

- This chapter will not be able to provide all the answers but hopefully it will provide sufficient stimulus to be of value in preparing for frailty in old age, with options for enjoying a quality of life based on the principles of choice, dignity and independence. Some of the key questions are:

- what are the options?
- what are realistic expectations of the care that will be available?
- will the state meet my needs?
- how much will it cost?
- who can provide me with answers?

Developing a strategy for an eventuality that may never happen, or may be five years or 25 years away, demands a broad-brush approach. Models of care are being developed all the time to suit the needs of a growing elderly population, with the state providing less care themselves, choosing instead to be purchasers of care and the elderly becoming "service users". Those delivering the care are called "providers". Although this terminology may have an impersonal ring, it is best to become *au fait* with it in order to be able successfully to navigate around the system. Market forces responding to a government set on reforming social policy are some of the more powerful influences on models of care provision. They remain, however, heavily influenced by the Treasury's grip on costs.

Whilst remaining at home is the preferred place for most people needing care, it is an expensive option. A service that is under-funded and, as a consequence,

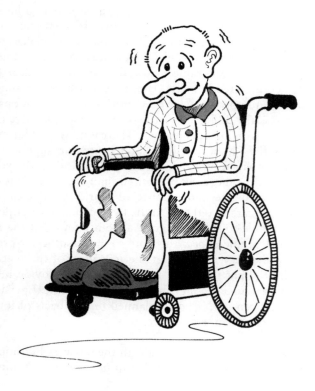

is based on the philosophy of minimum standards, may result in the vulnerable living in isolation, squalor and dependent on an aged spouse or friend as the principle carer. Most care options are not free but they are supported by state funding, which is subject to a financial means test. The positive aspect of the "purchaser/provider arrangement" is that older people now have purchasing power and a bewildering range of options available to them.

The guiding principle behind the level of provision of care services is to supply sufficient support to enable the individual to remain at home. The quality of life may be far from ideal and "unofficial" carers, such as partners and friends, may be expected to provide considerable support. Insufficient account is taken of the isolation, loneliness or sense of insecurity a vulnerable old person may feel. Ideally, the level of support should increase progressively in line with dependency until a point is reached when a care home with qualified staff is the best option to preserve the individual's quality of life.

The "care at home" services

This section covers all services that are provided in your own home, including practical support such as cleaning, meals, house repairs, shopping and befriending services. For the more dependent there is personal care including help with getting up and going to bed, toileting, bathing, washing, grooming and assistance with feeding. There is also a range of services for those individuals requiring nursing care that typically would include injections, administration of some drugs, dressing wounds and the management of more complex care packages.

These home delivered services are provided according to the current Social Services titles *Practical Support* and *Personal Care*. They are available to any individual but are only provided and funded by Social Services after a means test and are often in short supply. Typically the time allocated to a "client" is calculated in 15 minute slots, so the meagre resources are spread as thinly as possible. They are often delivered at times to suit a very busy schedule rather than at the person's preference. The level of expertise of the staff providing this service is expected to be equivalent to that which a caring relative should be able to provide. Charges are typically in the £4–8 per hour range for a care assistant although this figure varies enormously from the South to the North of England. The service is accessed through the Social Services Department. District Nurses provide nursing care at home; it is a free service and accessed through your GP.

Day care

Loneliness, isolation and becoming withdrawn from society may be reduced by attendance at a day care centre. These are often run by volunteer groups or by Social Services and provide a stimulating club-like atmosphere in which the day is organised around a programme of mental and physical activities, meals and the administration of treatment should any be needed. This service is an excellent way of giving a spouse or relative carer a break and some free time. Transport to and from the centre is sometimes provided. This service is means-tested and charges will include a contribution towards food. Charges are typically in the range £12–24 for a six-hour day. This may include the cost of lunch but transport would be an additional charge.

Supported housing

This generic term applies to a range of sheltered housing and housing with care models. They set out to provide the opportunity of independent living with the reassurance of assistance being available in case of an emergency. There are also many examples of housing for the frail who need a range of support and care. The accommodation on offer caters for a wide range of tastes, dependency levels and budgets. The standard sheltered housing schemes have a warden who answers the emergency call bell and organises an emergency response, but who is not necessarily permanently on site and may not be responsible for providing any practical support or care. They are now being replaced by warden-assisted schemes where some care is provided by the warden, and some provide an extensive range of caring services in-house.

Schemes such as Brendoncare's *Close Care* housing scheme at Alton, Hampshire makes available a level of support to the individual at home equivalent to that provided in a residential or nursing home. The apartments are located in the grounds of a nursing home and the emergency call system is manned by staff 24 hours a day. On-call carers provide a response service 365 days a year. The home acts as a resource centre for the *Close Care* residents, providing in addition to nursing care, a licensed restaurant, hairdressing salon, library and shop. Other useful services such as a handyman, gardener, laundry and shopping service are also available. There is a standard service charge to cover property maintenance and "warden" services, with all other services charged on a per item of service basis. This type of provision is increasingly seen as the alternative to residential care.

Charges for these services are difficult to summarise. The housing element may be offered for rent, lease, or sale. The service element, that should include the warden service, will vary according to the range of services supplied.

Residential and nursing care

Since April 2002 both residential and nursing homes are now known collectively as care homes. However, the level of dependency in any care home is determined by staffing skills and levels, the environment and facilities. It can be difficult and confusing for the prospective service users to determine whether a particular group of needs can be met in a care home.

The need for residential or nursing care in a care home is usually determined by a multidisciplinary team assessment by Health and Social Service representatives. It is possible to access these services directly if the state is not expected to support the fees. The criteria for admission to a care home are based on whether the individual is able to live independently at home. The availability of support from relatives and community care services and the economical cost of remaining at home are taken into account. The choice and wishes of the service user regarding their preferred care home have to be taken into account and should the individual without an adequate occupational pension have wealth of less than £19,000 (the 2002 figure, which is reviewed annually) the state will begin to provide financial support for fees.

This service is means-tested and regulated by the National Care Standards Commission. A statutory framework exists within this sector and by virtue of its prescriptive nature defines the services available. It aims to provide community living where quality care homes ensure that care is individualised and personal choice is reflected in the care plan and the way each day is organised.

A care home is required to have an experienced and qualified manager, but if there are no qualified nurses on site, nursing care is provided via the district nursing service. The level of care the home is expected to deliver is set out in 38 care standards. A summary of these should be available from the home together with their "Statement of Purpose". This document sets out the range of services available and the approach to looking after the individual. For example, it should contain details of staffing levels which are the key to being able to provide good care.

There is no short cut to selecting a suitable home. It is probably one of the last major decisions of one's life and ranks alongside buying a house in terms of the possible financial commitment and related stress levels. Below are a few tips to help with this exercise.

Choosing a care home

For most people choosing a care home is outside their experience and they respond by using the same criteria as for choosing a hotel. This approach tends to place undue emphasis on the facilities available and does not address the type of care, quality and appropriateness of the service. There is no substitute for personal viewing but visiting many care homes can present major logistical problems, especially as the "service user" is likely to be too frail to participate and requires a spouse, relative or friend to make the decision. A four stage approach is suggested as a guide:

1. Define the criteria

Produce a list of the essential and desirable features you expect to see in the home, e.g. location, size, single room, ensuite bathroom, nursing care available, specialist nursing equipment such as hoists, assisted bathrooms, good food, like-minded company.

2. Research

Obtain a full list of homes from the Social Services Department in the area in which you wish to live. It will contain details of the level of care available, e.g. for low- to medium-dependency, a residential home which does not have qualified nursing staff would be suitable. For higher dependency, a nursing home with qualified nursing staff on duty at all times would be more appropriate.

- Select a list of around 6–9 homes based on your criteria.
- Obtain from each home all their literature and information including website address if they have one.
- Obtain from the homes their last two (or more) inspection reports.
- From all the information gathered compare each home with your criteria and select a shortlist of 2 or 3 homes to visit.
- Arrange a viewing appointment with a senior representative of each home.

3. Viewing and selection

Before the visit do your homework – prepare a list of questions arising from the literature and the inspection reports.

To avoid sensory overload, have a plan of approach, this apt acronym may help:

F facilities
A approach or philosophy of care
E experience of staff
C care standards
E expense and fees
S suitability, will the individual fit in?

- Upon arrival be honest about the needs of the individual you are seeking to place.
- Expect to be given a tour, but it is an individual's home, so access may be restricted.
- View the room on offer, note its size, the furnishings, room aspect, view details of ensuite facilities, distance from the main socialising areas. Many homes will allow residents to have their own furniture.
- View the public areas: sitting rooms, dining room, activities room etc. to make sure they are comfortable and suitable.
- Visit the service areas: you will probably not be allowed into the kitchen for valid environmental health reasons but view as much as possible – the state of repair and tidiness may give a valuable insight into how well the home is organised.
- Discuss with the manager or matron the inspection reports and any issues arising from them plus other questions arising from the literature or the visit. Ask for a copy of the resident's contract and terms of admission.
- Enquire about a trial visit, perhaps for a day or even a week. The home is required to offer this so you are not asking them a favour, but expect to pay for this service.

4. Decision

By this stage you will have a good idea of which home suits your needs best, the availability of a bedroom, costs and timescale.

If you are still unsure, revisit but this time ask to meet some staff and, if possible, some of the residents. Raise with them some of the questions that may still be unanswered in your mind. The best homes will use this as an opportunity to demonstrate how central residents are in their approach to care.

Costs

The figures in Table 1 are for guidance only as there are regional variances for both Social Service grants and independent sector charges.

Table 1 Current fee levels (April 2002) – for London add £70 approx. per week

	Social Service Grant (£ per week)	ACO* (£ per week)	Private (£ per week)
Residential care	225	340	400+
Nursing home	336–425	490	500–750

*Association of Charity Officers' published recommended rate

From these figures care in a low-dependency home would typically cost in the region of £11,700–20,800 per annum. In a high-dependency home the range would typically be from £17,500–39,000 per annum. The top end of the fee scale is usually for the more specialist homes caring for the mentally ill with physical needs. However, just like choosing a hotel, luxurious care is available at a higher price.

Further information

Health and social care professionals are the gatekeepers of the majority of services for older people. Social workers manage the grants system and local authority Social Service departments co-ordinate the assessment process.

Under legislation introduced in April 2002, providers of care in care homes are obliged to provide details of the most recent Care Standards Commission inspection reports, and to produce a comprehensive description of the services they provide in a document called a "Statement of Purpose" in addition to regular surveys of their service users to measure "customer satisfaction". The domicillary care sector will be similarly regulated by the end of 2002.

- The National Care Standards Commission helpline is 0191 233 3556 and their website is www.carestandards.org.uk.
- The Citizens' Advice Bureaux can provide a list of care homes.
- Association of Charity Officers provides advice on "top up grants"; telephone: 01707 651777 fax: 01707 660477
- Help the Aged provide a free welfare rights advice line *SeniorLine* 0808 800 6565 and their website, www.helptheaged.org.uk provides a range of free advice sheets on all aspects of residential care.
- The Brendoncare Foundation provides care homes for the physically and mentally ill, *Close Care* sheltered housing and "care at home" schemes. For further details telephone 01962 852133 or visit their website www.brendoncare.org.uk

RS

CHAPTER 18

Depression and mental adjustments in retirement

Why should retirement make me depressed?

Retirement does not come very high on the list of life events precipitating depressive illness. Bereavement, physical illness and even moving house are far more important events which can be felt as losses, but retirement brings its own set of changes:

- the end of full-time occupation
- the loss of such status as attaches to one's employment, and change to that of senior citizen or pensioner
- loss of company of colleagues
- reduction in income
- reduced life expectancy
- more time at home, either alone or with one's partner.

Loss of occupation

The end of full-time occupation is a serious loss for "workaholics" and those with few outside interests. Their *raison d'être* seems to have gone when they are no longer required to work. Doctors in particular have led busy lives, often absorbed by their job. I recall the story of a salesman who on reaching the age of 65 was required to cease working and give back his company car. Only then did he face the finality of his employment. On his bewildered walk home he passed the gates of a mental hospital and sought emergency asylum from the alarm and despondency which were making him suddenly suicidal. With the loss of occupation may come the loss of a full, structured working day. Some will relish this but others may wonder "What on earth am I going to do with myself?"

Loss of status

The loss of status is felt keenly by those who need their professional standing to sustain their self-confidence. The days of Richard Gordon's character, Sir Lancelot Spratt, with his entourage of subservient junior doctors, nurses and students, bellowing "You must pursue me!" as he bore down on his awe-struck patients, may be past but some doctors may miss power and prestige, their authority in the theatre, ward rounds, clinic or the surgery and being needed and in demand.

The transition to senior citizen may seem degrading, especially to those who have mocked or despised "geriatrics" throughout their clinical careers. "Senior citizen" sounds a bit grander than "old age pensioner" but they are one and the same. Senior citizens are entitled to free travel on London Transport, and discounts using Senior Railcards, and get concessionary prices in theatres, galleries and cinemas but such citizenship may be perceived as belonging to a dependant, rather too large minority of elders, and even on a continuum with the despised and resented "bed-blockers", burdening and obstructing an over-stretched NHS.

> I grow old … I grow old …
> I shall wear the bottoms of my trousers rolled.
> TS Eliot *The Love Song of J. Alfred Prufrock*

Loss of company

The loss of the company of colleagues is particularly important to those who have few other friendships and my not be good at making friends. Those who have commuted to work will have had limited opportunities to get to know people in their own community, and may at first feel somewhat stranded after retirement.

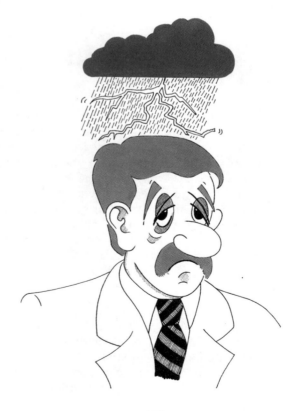

Loss of earnings

The lump sum received on retirement is very welcome, but subsequently the monthly income is noticeably less than during working life, and anxieties about a reduced lifestyle may be an unpleasant preoccupation. The provident 'ants', with their 'added years' and well-managed savings, will be at an advantage here over the carefree, live-for-the-moment 'grasshoppers' who have never taken seriously the idea that they might live beyond 65 and trust to the gods that somehow they will be taken care of thereafter.

> Drink and dance and laugh and lie,
> Dance the reeling midnight through;
> For tomorrow we may die
> (But, alas, we never do!)'
>
> Dorothy Parker

Reduced life expectancy

Reduced life expectancy is rarely a specific consequence of retirement, through one is anecdotally aware of some dedicated doctors whose abrupt deaths within months of that event suggested that they could not live without their work. Retirement is, however, one of those significant milestones, like the 40th, 60th and 70th birthdays, which is accompanied by an appreciation of the limitations of mortality.

> The days of our years are three score and ten; and though some men be so strong that they come to four score years, yet is their strength then but labour and sorrow; so soon passeth it away and they are gone.
>
> Psalm 90, v 10

After retirement one is liable to read the obituary columns in *The Times* and the *British Medical Journal* more closely and to take particular note of the birth dates of those who have passed on, and still more of the deaths of one's contemporaries which become ever more frequent.

> *Eheu, figaces, Postume, Postume*
> *Labuntur anni.*
>
> Horace. Odes, bk 2, no.14.1.1

More time at home

It may seem unduly cynical to regard what many would consider a bonus as a loss, but for those who live alone there is the threat of loneliness and for those who live with another there is the problem of being too much together to be negotiated, "I married him for better or for worse – but not for lunch!" Marital tension may increase for a while after retirement as couples, used only to spending all day together at weekends or on holiday, find that this is a life-sentence! Some may simply dread a loss of privacy and personal space.

If retirement is followed by depression it may in part be due to one or some of the above. However, most people enter retirement equably, or even embrace it eagerly, as a time for leisure and pursuing personal interests. Depression at this time is particularly associated with

- a past history of depression
- unwanted retirement, on the grounds of ill health or, rarely, redundancy
- personal illness, or that of one's partner
- poverty (unusual, we hope, among doctors!)
- marital discord.

The symptoms of depression in retirement

Depression may actually be a cause of seeking early retirement. So-called "burn-out' may be a manifestation of depressive illness, and the decision to retire may be ill-judged; important decisions are best avoided while one is seriously depressed. Relief from the pressures of work may be followed by misgivings about having given up without finishing the job and the prospect of a dwindling future ("I couldn't stand the heat, so I had to get out of the kitchen", or "I had such high hopes when I qualified, it's all ended in frustration and failure".). In depressive illness the power of negative thinking is especially potent.

> Tomorrow, and tomorrow, and tomorrow,
> Creeps in this pretty pace from day to day
> To the last syllable of recorded time,
> And all our yesterdays have lighted fools
> The way to dusty death.
>
> Shakespeare, *Macbeth* Act V, Sc 5

Doctors are not especially good at recognising depression in themselves. It is not easy to stand back from one's clinical disorder. Doctors are by no means immune to the stigma which is attached to psychiatric disorders and may be reluctant to concede that they could be depressed. However enlightened and compassionate they may have been in dealing with their patients, when they weigh themselves in balance they may find themselves wanting, "Depression is for wimps."

Even if there have been previous spells of depression, successfully treated, there can be great difficulty in acknowledging that it is happening again. Even with insight there can be difficulty in seeking and finding help. "Who can I go to who won't think less of me? If I go to my own GP it'll be all over town in a week or two... I suppose I could write myself a prescription for an antidepressant, but which one? What about side-effects? Do they really work? Not for quite a while, I've been told. Perhaps I ought to see a psychiatrist – or a psychologist – but who can I trust? Who's any good?" All doctors are somewhat at risk of being treated as "special" by their colleagues: there are hazards of over-investigation and treatment on one hand, and a breezy "you know all this so what would you like me to do?" approach on the other.

Symptoms suggestive of depressive illness include:

- loss of interests and enjoyment of life (anhedonia)
- lack of drive and motivation – "can't be bothered" "too much effort".
- loss of confidence
- introversion
- loss of affectionate feelings, going off sex
- dithering and indecision
- anxiety and irritability
- guilt and loss of self-esteem
- misery and pessimism ("gloom and doom")
- forgetfulness (due to mental slowing and anxious, depressed preoccupation) which may be morbidly ascribed to a degenerative disease such as Alzheimer's
- suicidal thoughts
- utter fatigue
- loss of appetite and loss of weight (or occasionally "comfort eating" and weight gain)
- insomnia, especially in the small hours
- feeling worse in the first half of the day.

There may have been a clear onset or exacerbation of these symptoms within recent weeks or months, and quality of life and social functioning are markedly impaired.

Preventing depression in retirement

Primary prevention

We cannot alter our heredity or early upbringing. Risk factors for depression such as maternal deprivation in childhood are beyond our control. If we are a cyclothymic personality, with mood swings, we may have found the energy and creativity of our upswings advantageous, though soldiering through the depressive downturns is an effort. If we are serious and obsessional, those traits may have been assets in our career, yet render us more liable to get depressed under stress.

Given that we are what we are, how can we render ourselves less likely to suffer depression as we retire and get older?

1. *Mens sana in corpore sano*
If we don't neglect our health we are less likely to suffer those maladies which blight life. Stroke, myocardial infarction, chronic obstructive airway disease and fractured femur are particularly depressing disorders, so watching diet, weight, blood pressure, cholesterol and taking enough exercise are important. Cycling, swimming, golf and dog walking (but don't fall over the dog!) are good forms of exercise in later life, though some diehards will continue to be active in the gym, on the tennis court and climb mountains. Few doctors have

the resolve to carry on smoking in the face of peer disapproval, but those who do so will pay the price in heart and lung disease as they get older. Alcohol, on the other hand, especially Chilean Cabernet Sauvignon, seems to be positively beneficial in moderation.

2. *Don't stop work all at once*

Most doctors know when they could, should or must retire and may be able to ease their workload before the actual day. This allows time to explore leisure opportunities and other interests and get to know better the neighbourhood in which they live. Again, many doctors have the opportunity of taking some part-time remunerative employment after they officially retire, which means that they don't stop work altogether but do less. Medico-legal work can create a new and rewarding interest as one grapples with the law and its very different view of illness and injury. Full-time locum posts bring in the money for those who badly need it, and while they may also bring in work stress one is largely relieved of administrative responsibilities.

3. *Promote your interests*

If you are already a committed lepidopterist or astronomer with a necessary interest in medicine retirement will liberate you to do what you love most. If, on the other hand you approach retirement with no other strings to your bow than medicine you will feel bereft as opportunities to practise your art dwindle. So it behoves you to foster outside interests, be they scientific, charitable, literary, artistic, political, religious, historical, horticultural, theatrical – whatever. Doctors are bright and well-educated and have a duty to diversify and make the widest use of their talents. Their reward is to see retirement as an opportunity, not a restriction.

4. *Cherish your personal relationships*

In retirement you may make fewer new friends, but may consolidate longer standing relationships. Marriage is foremost among these and needs to be worked at: you and your spouse will be spending more time together than ever before, and if things aren't good they can be abysmally bad. Sex is "90% of the problem but 10% of the answer" but well worth sustaining, even into the seventh age! Grandchildren are a greater bonus than their parents, and you might even come to like your neighbours.

5. *Enjoy your leisure*

You can now discover the joys of afternoon television, particularly the nostalgia of those old films and the quiz shows: you might even be a contender on *Fifteen to One*. Now is an excellent time to have longer holidays, take a cruise or possibly move to that place in the country or by the sea which you've cherished over the years. You can catch up with your reading – Proust or *War and Peace* can still be conquered before you die. Crosswords, Scrabble and bridge are fun and help to keep your brain active.

Secondary prevention

The earlier the recognition, acknowledgement and treatment of depression the sooner it is over and the less its ill-effects. Getting help means overcoming passive nihilism and perhaps swallowing pride. Whatever misgivings one may have about competence and confidentiality, the GP is likely to be the best key to appropriate help in the first instance. He or she may start treatment or may call upon mental health specialists like the psychiatrist, psychologist or community psychiatric nurse.

Antidepressant drugs work better than placebo. Though the serotonin-specific reuptake inhibitors (SSRIs) have largely replaced the tricyclics, whose anticholinergic side-effects are generally less well tolerated, it appears that venlafaxine [a serotonin and noradrenaline reuptake inhibitor (SNRI)] may currently be the most effective antidepressant. Antidepressants must, of course, be taken in sufficient dosage: it is no kindness to a colleague to prescribe "a small dose in case it should help" except for the placebo effect. Benzodiazepines have had a particularly "bad press" but a small dose of lorazepam (1 mg) can be very useful in easing anxiety until the antidepressant "kicks in".

For those who dislike the idea of medication, or "pills for personal problems", talking treatments have greater appeal. Simply off-loading to a detached but sympathetic listener can be immediately beneficial, and further counselling from such a person provides valuable support and encouragement, not least that there is light at the end of the tunnel. If there are marital problems counselling is especially useful, from *RELATE* for example. Psychotherapy is usually dynamic, uncovering suppressed hostility, for example, and using transference – the feelings the patient develops for the therapist – as a way of exploration and gaining insight. It may be very beneficial in helping one cope with the sort of situations which have brought on depression in the past, but is hard to handle while one is severely depressed. Overall, the evidence most strongly supports cognitive behavioural therapy (CBT) which addresses the negative thinking intrinsic to depression and stresses which appears to trigger gloom, over the course of 12–16 sessions of 50 minutes. It seems that combining antidepressant therapy and CBT is especially potent.

Tertiary prevention

There is a great temptation to stop treatment, particularly medication, before it has had time to work ("Oh, this is useless – I knew it would be") or as soon as well-being starts to return ("Great, I'm almost OK – now it's up to me!"). Knowing too much about the different classes of antidepressants can lead to disastrous chopping and changing before any have been taken long enough, while relief at beginning to feel all right again leads to premature withdrawal from therapy. Antidepressants should be taken for at least six months after full recovery, and indefinitely where there has been improvement but some residual symptoms (e.g. early walking, dysphoria for an hour or two after rising) continue. Where lithium has been prescribed (for bipolar affective disorder or for resistant depression) it is particularly important to "keep taking the tablets".

Counselling and CBT require some effort on the patient's part, but persistence pays dividends.

Those who appear to have seasonal affective disorder (SAD), and find their spirits lower as the day lengths shorten, may find prolonged exposure to sun lamps, 4–5 hours per day, helpful. Having a pet which needs attention (mammalian preferred!) helps to keep one going despite depression, and may even hasten recovery.

Self help

If you are depressed you need the help of professional others, but there are some ways in which you can help yourself:

- Do something to break depressive apathy and inertia – change a light bulb, pay a bill, answer a letter, empty a wastepaper basket. You will feel that at least you have accomplished something and are not completely useless.
- Take some exercise, enough to make you sweat – go for a walk, a jog, dig the garden. There's evidence that regular exercise has some antidepressant effect and it's also good for your general health and may help you to sleep better.
- If you can't sleep don't toss and turn but get up (trying not to disturb your partner), go to another room and read, watch a video, listen to music until you are dozing off, then go back to bed.
- Make sure you eat enough even if you lack appetite: fresh fruit and vegetables are recommended. You may care to try St John's Wort (hypericum) daily which works as an antidepressant for those who are mildly depressed.
- Moderate alcohol intake is compatible with antidepressant therapy, but beware of "drowning your sorrows" especially if you have had problems with alcohol in the past.
- Try to remind yourself that you are going through a bad phase but it will pass: like fog, night-time and winter, depression is a self-limiting disorder.

> Grow old along with me! The best is yet to be,
> The last of life for which the first was made:
> Our times are in his hand who says 'A whole I planned
> Youth knows but half; trust God, see all: nor be afraid!
>
> Robert Browning *Rabbi Ben Ezra*, st 1
>
> BP

Further reading

- *Coping with Loss* edited by Colin Murray Parkes and Andres Markus: BMJ Books, London.
- *Darkness Visible* by William Styron: Jonathan Cape. London.
- *Depression and How to Survive It* by Spike Milligan and Anthony Clare: Edbury Press, London.
- *Down With Gloom* by Brice Pitt and Mel Calman: Gaskell Press, London.

- *Malignant Sadness: the anatomy of depression* by Lewis Wolpert: Faber and Faber, London.
- *An Unquiet Mind* by Kay Redfield Jamieson: Picador, London.

Useful addresses

- Depression Alliance, 35 Westminster Bridge Road, London SE1 7JB; telephone: 0207 633 0557; website: www.depressionalliance.org
- RELATE, Herbert Gray College, Little Church Street, Rugby CV21 3AP; telephone: 01788 573 241
- Royal College of Psychiatrists (External Affairs), 17 Belgrave Square, London SW1X 8PG; telephone: 020 7235 2351; website: www.rcpsych.org.uk
- The Samaritans; Helpline 08457 909090; textphone: 08457 909192; website: www.samaritans.org.uk

(Information correct May 2002)

CHAPTER 19

Bereavement

There are two inevitable consequences of reaching retirement age. The first, that one will lose a close relative or friend, and the second is that one will die. Both may be helped with foresight and, where possible, with preparation. We cannot prepare for sudden death in an accident or from an acute illness, but, by retiring age the likelihood of dying has already been present for some years and, therefore, some thought may be helpful.

Most sensible people do prepare at least partially for death in a practical way, by disposing of assets, making a will, and deciding what possessions should go to whom. That is not at all the same thing as emotional preparation for death. The first book in this series, *A Career in Medicine: do you have what it takes?* prepares students to enter medicine, with an apparently boundless future ahead of them. This book is totally different, aimed at doctors finishing their career, at a time when one is faced with preparation for a more finite future concluding with one's own death.

This chapter will not deal with the practicalities of making wills and disposing of one's possessions – these tasks are discussed in another chapter. I aim to deal in a helpful way with the emotional consequences of the death of family and friends. This is a subject that most people dislike contemplating for fairly obvious reasons and, unless there has been a long period of illness, the final days arrive without any proper preparation for death.

The process of grieving

Being bereaved means facing a whole series of different emotions and novel tasks, for which there can be some preparation. Grief can certainly occur before death takes place, sometimes with the person who will depart, and may be therapeutic for both parties. A wonderful example of this and how to cope with grief is to be found in the book by C S Lewis, *A Grief Observed* (Faber and Faber, London). Lewis was a Catholic theologian, an academic and a wonderful observer and writer. He lived from 1898 to 1963, marrying Joy Davidman in 1956. She died of cancer in 1960. He grieved with his wife when she had been diagnosed with cancer, and they spent much time discussing the future. When he realised that he would have to be separated by death from his wife, he started recording his observations on the grief that they were suffering and sharing together. His observations and feelings are exceptionally well-observed and honest. A major part of his published version recounts his memories of their discussions, and their individual attitudes to her death. Lewis describes what he thinks grief actually is and how he and his wife were affected by it before her death. The worst thing about death for them and for many other couples was the forthcoming separation that had to be suffered. Their life together had given them both so much pleasure that there was great pain in contemplating this loss of companionship.

Lewis' book it is not a sad book and the account of their companionship in marriage will be an inspiration to all happily married couples. It was written with such empathy and sympathy that in various forms it has had an enormous readership – it was reprinted many times, and adapted as the play *Shadowlands* which also enjoyed great success as a film. The book, the play and the film strike a chord with many people who have suffered the same deprivation. It is so highly thought of that *CRUSE*, a professional organisation formed to help the bereaved, places Lewis' book, play and film as their first recommendation for reading during bereavement.

A second book recommended by *CRUSE*, *Living With Grief* (Sheldon Press, London), is written by Dr Tony Lake, a psychotherapist and accredited counsellor of the British Association of Counselling. He has defined grief as "something you do, not something which happens to you". It is an active process, which may take time to develop. He says, "you can only successfully carry out each of the tasks of your own grief when you are ready to do so". We have to accept some of the changes that are to occur, but not all of them at once.

Bereavement is not the same as grief, although it certainly may lead to grief. There is a need to adapt to the death of a loved one. It can have substantial physiological consequences which may be mild or severe. Grief almost always brings tiredness, partly due to sleep disturbance which is quite normal, as is some loss of appetite and associated weight loss. Sleep may be completely distorted with bad dreams and only achieved after tossing and turning in bed thinking of the death. Occasionally sleep will contain good dreams of the time spent with the lost one or one may wake up every day thinking of the lost one or the day they first heard of the death. Recent articles in the *British Medical Journal* reveal that there are definite biochemical abnormalities that occur with deep grief. Yet life has to continue, and these symptoms may lessen but are not likely to disappear completely for weeks or even months.

It is not a continuous or steady progression. At first, there may be so much shock at the death of the loved one that overt mourning hardly makes any appearance at all. Instead, a bemused, shocked state takes over. Gradually, however, a different feeling will develop and strangely enough it may be an absolute emptiness for a few weeks or months, to be followed by subsequent mood-swings. And then, months or even years later, something may trigger a different stage of the mourning process. Everyone mourns in a different way and every part of mourning is different. Eventually, acceptance of the loss dominates and then, in most cases, the mourner may not find it necessary ever to return to the states experienced at the beginning. There is hope at the end of the tunnel and gradually the grief may become less deep or it may be episodic before it dies out.

Lake also says of the grieving process, "Many [mourners] resist fixed ideas and expectations and the habits of others." I myself do not think that anyone should be forced to do what is expected by others even when grieving. For instance, fifty years or so ago, mourning required dark clothes, wearing black ties and looking mournful. But the process of mourning has changed within the space of a couple of generations and the outside trappings of mourning do not have to be worn. They may have been very helpful some decades back but today do very little for the mourner.

While it is not necessary to advertise one's grief, it is very helpful to have someone to share it. Grief in older people who are retired is often followed by isolation. It is important to recognise that independence is vital and that building a new future without the companionship of the dead person is essential. Isolation is not inevitable and help in many circumstances can be very valuable. Each person feels his or her loss differently. The greatest grief of all may arise with returning to the home that had been shared with the deceased. Coming home may be very distressing every day. You may automatically shout out "I'm home" and this can be intensely sad because inevitably there is no reply. It is helpful to have confidence in one's own inner strengths to cope with this feeling. Such qualities have previously got one through other trials and tribulations in life. "Time", says Lake, "does not heal, but it does have a therapeutic quality in grief."

Often some very strange emotions bubble up after bereavement. One woman could not get over what she felt to be the selfishness of her husband who died before she did. "How could he do this to me?" she said, "We had so much to live for together in our retirement." This illustrates why loss in early retirement can be much worse than loss during an active career. Anger against the dead person is not an uncommon phenomenon and it is understandable, because in dying they have inevitably caused deprivation.

A much more common emotion is guilt, "If only we had done this" or "If only I had taken more notice of what she was saying". Of course, the guilt is worse if one feels responsible for the death such as in a motor accident. Even when there is no obvious responsibility people still feel guilty. You may not feel guilty for causing the death but may feel guilty for any disagreements which may have lessened the quality of life of the deceased, "If only we had not had a row".

Although Lake's book is full of explanations that can help in many ways, I would recommend it with caution to someone who believes that they are beginning to cope with their loss without external help. Too much analysis may bring out additional elements of the grief and instead of helping may make adjustment more difficult.

Letters

When people hear or read that someone has died, they often sit down to write a letter of condolence. These letters are not easy to write, and in some circumstances, such as suicide, may be so difficult that people just do not write. They explain this by saying, "I sat down to write, but I just did not know what to say." A letter thought out carefully can be of great comfort, but one that has not been thought out carefully may do just the opposite. A good letter may provoke an outburst of crying, which is not necessarily a bad thing and it does not lessen the comfort given by the letter.

Probably the most comforting letters are those that extol the virtues of the deceased, giving the mourner pride in the relationship that existed with the dead person. This is especially so if the writer emphasizes that memories of the dead person involve significant achievements, valued by society, as is often the case with doctors.

However, there are letters that are not helpful. So many letters seem to be themselves cries for help by the writer, who states that they have been through a bereavement, "I know exactly how you feel". I suspect this may actually mean, "I know that I am suffering and quite possibly you are suffering like me, but I do need support in my suffering – can we get together and share this?" This may appear selfish and unfeeling to the reader even though it was not intended that way.

Well-intentioned but unspecific suggestions may be unhelpful. "Please let me know what I can do for you" is not much use unless accompanied by a positive offer such as, "I would like to take you out for a meal". It is even better when it suggests a definite date. Anything vague like "Do let me know when you would like to go to the theatre with me" is clearly not very helpful – it is much better to be practical, "If you feel like it, I would like to take you out. I will phone you in a few days' time to suggest some arrangements."

Of course everybody's suffering is different. It is not possible to know exactly how the person to whom you are writing is feeling at the moment when they read your letter. Mourning is a process that occurs day by day, with its ups and downs and this may go on for a long time. The mourning may be quite different at the end of a month or two than that felt six months later. Great care, therefore, should be taken when writing the condolence letter. It is polite to acknowledge every single letter and message, if only with a printed reply. You may naturally feel a temptation to add something personal to the formal acknowledgement and this is no doubt appreciated by the recipient. When acknowledging a letter of condolence do not dwell too much on your own losses or troubles.

Music

Many people find listening to music the greatest consolation of all, and particularly helpful may be listening to music that has been enjoyed together with the deceased, or even a journey with music that has been enjoyed together. Seeing Fingal's Cave on a cruise around the Scottish Islands brought back to me the memories of a concert performance of the piece which proved very touching indeed.

Memorials

The Taj Mahal, the 17th century mausoleum near Agra, India was built by the Emperor Shah Jahan in memory of his wife who died in childbirth after nineteen years of marriage. It is probably the world's greatest memorial and declaration of love. Unfortunately, we cannot all build such commemorative buildings but we can in much smaller ways create lasting memorials. Of course, as many churches throughout the country show, traditionally people have chosen memorial tablets or statues. A popular memorial to be found in many parks is a bench inscribed with the name of the deceased. Alternatively, many theatres and concert halls also offer the opportunity to name a seat in their auditorium. A larger and more productive memorial is to plant a tree, create a garden or even a whole wood. This form of commemoration is becoming more popular. Visiting such a garden or wood can be therapeutic for the mourner. Any such constructive forms of commemoration that can grow or even protect a piece of nature from neglect or development can be a beneficial memorial.

Prolonging one's presence is also possible with a professional memorial reflecting one's work and achievements in life, such as a scholarship for needy students. However, I would advise against eponymous lectures because they can be an enormous headache to administer and the subject after whom the lecture is named will almost certainly be forgotten within a decade, making it difficult to attract audiences.

Getting help in bereavement

Tony Lake says, "We have to accept what is going to happen or what happens and very often have to get help from other people." These may be grieving with us and those with whom we share our lives. Most people naturally turn to members of their own family for consolation and support, but they may be equally weakened and upset by the loss and not be in a position to help. Although mourning together as a family has long been recognised as a very helpful form of mourning, it is not always the most practical. There are now professional organisations that help by enabling people to understand their grief and cope with their loss. *CRUSE* is just one organisation, with over 160 local branches, that have been set up to help the bereaved. It does so not only by recommending books, but also by arranging meetings and lectures and literature that will be helpful. It will also provide somebody who has been trained to talk to a bereaved person and who meets the sufferer face-to-face and talks in confidence.

The Samaritans provide emotional support with someone to talk to over the telephone 24 hours every day of the week and they also offer over 200 local walk-in centres if you prefer to discuss things face-to-face with someone. There are many websites dealing with the subject, offering discussion groups and advice. Further details for bereavement resources are given at the end of this chapter.

Planning for the future

After operations patients appear to get well more quickly if they can set themselves targets for recovery. Grief can be seen as an illness from which recovery will take place, but recovery may be helped with certain positive steps such as taking up a new interest or by continuing to excel in a worthwhile daily

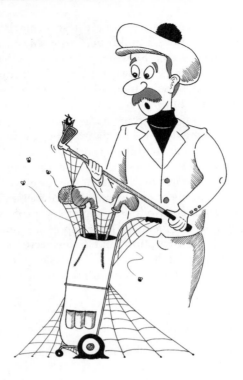

occupation such as work. But in retirement, daily work and the satisfaction of doing it may well have been taken away, so it is constructive and indeed helpful to look for a new hobby or to work at something creative like playing a musical instrument, painting or maybe getting your old golf clubs out and taking some lessons. After all, Grandma Moses (Anna Mary Robertson Moses) was a widow in her late seventies before she took up painting very successfully. Bridge has been said by many widows to be their salvation because it has two ends – it is first an excuse to mix with other people of a similar age and situation, and it is also a satisfying intellectual challenge.

Nobody can set a pattern for anybody else as to how to grieve successfully nor how to overcome grief, but there are a number of helpful organisations – some of which are listed below.

EP

Further information

- CRUSE Bereavement Care, Cruse House, 126 Sheen Road, Richmond, Surrey TW9 1UR; "Day-by-day" helpline: 0870 167 1677; website www.crusebereavementcare.org.uk
- National Association of Bereavement Services (NABS) can give advice about local bereavement services: NABS, 20 Norton Folgate, London E1 6DB; helpline: 020 7247 0617 (answered weekdays 10 am–4 pm)

- National Association of Widows, National Office, 48 Queens Road, Coventry CV1 3EH; helpline: 024 7663 4848 (answerphone at times)
- *Retirement Matters* website, www.retirement-matters.co.uk, carries a particularly useful article written by GP Dr David Delvin about bereavement.
- The Royal College of Psychiatrists' website offers several resources, in particular:
  Bereavement Information Pack for those bereaved suddenly or by suicide: www.rcpsych.ac.uk/publications.gaskell/bereav
  Bereavement Fact sheet:
  www.rcpsych.ac.uk/info/help/bereav/index.htm
- The Samaritans; telephone: 08457 909090; textphone: 08457 909192; website: www.samaritans.org.uk

(Information correct May 2002)

CHAPTER 20

Religion and death

*R*eligion for most of us will be a rather personal and private matter. Some may have discarded formal beliefs and practices in the course of a demanding professional life – and even questioned the relevance in adult life of childhood indoctrination in such matters. The historical fact is that the religion we inherited by a biological chance of parenthood has largely dictated the structure of our lives. This includes both education and apprenticeship in our professional years. Somehow the way in which we have cared for our patients will, even subconsciously, have been influenced by the spiritual discipline and ethical concepts offered to us when we were young. What else fostered our vocation and underpinned our endeavours to heal and maintain a good quality of life in our patients? Whom did we admire from our formative years and seek to emulate? We might even begin to wonder what in their own time influenced our teachers and, in turn, what we have passed on to our families, friends and the juniors who have worked with us in the past.

A sense of eternity and our relationship with it becomes ever more relevant in our retiring years. We cannot escape revisiting this aspect of our existence, even if it has been previously discarded for some years. We may discard it once more but we owe a certain amount of introspection both to ourselves and those around us in deciding how we will now conduct our lives in retirement. Perhaps we can confirm the values which we believe to be important in our own lives and the direction in which we wish to continue. We might even address any defects which we identify! This I believe is our duty and it is this which led me to solicit the following short non-denominational post-script to our professional lives when we contemplate our retirement, our demise and our place in eternity.

Ed

When thought is given to retirement in the 21st century, it must be considered in relation to the massive changes that have occurred in the world of work in recent times. In the past, people's work occurred within fairly rigid structures. Many remained with one company or institution for the whole of their working lives, gradually moving up the hierarchy. The customs, patterns and relationships of their institutions were almost an extended family and retirement would naturally result in a feeling of exclusion or loss.

A friend of mine who had lived all of his working life within such an environment described his retirement as though he had been travelling in a bus filled with all his best friends in a party atmosphere when suddenly the vehicle stops, everyone waves goodbye and the lighted bus moves on leaving him alone by the road-side. The world of work is now very different. People often change their occupations many times in their careers and even those who remain within one institution or one profession have to adapt to massive changes. The educational world that I entered in 1962 had totally changed by the time I left it in 1992. Consequently, people have to live more diverse and flexible lives.

Men are nowadays experiencing what has been a previously typical female career path, involving learning the pleasures of housework, cookery and child (or grandchild-) care. I know two women who married upon leaving university and spent a number of years caring for their family, returning to their professional careers in their forties. One became a senior civil servant and the other a professor. For many families it is not always the mother who makes the "career sacrifice" and it is more and more acceptable for fathers to excel as a "house-husband". Some may argue that this affects men's self-esteem, that they are reluctant to give up their position as the major earner in the household but experience is proving that men can be equally successful and equally valued as their female counterparts when spending several years away from full-time work in their role as home-makers.

All this adaptation makes the experience of retirement less traumatic than it was in the past. If one has learnt flexibility and adaptability during a full-time working life, it is possible to use these skills within one's retirement. The change need not be as abrupt as it was in the past. The fact is that because of changes in working practices, the "full-time" job is no longer the whole sum of life – many attractive and suitable vacancies are available to people not in full time employment. Voluntary occupations like the Citizens Advice Bureaux, school chaperoning, education committees, parish councils to name but a few can result in a wide variety of useful and interesting tasks to perform. To return to the bus metaphor – there are lots of other buses waiting.

However, retirement or the reduction in full-time work is also associated with old age. The adage that "old age is not for cissies" becomes ever more true as we experience the illnesses and weaknesses that are an integral part of the ageing process. Inevitably, one considers the fact of death – here again, it is important to consider life as a seamless whole and not to divide it into compartments. In the past it has been the practice to regard working life as a time of activity, when one admittedly did one's religious duties, and only in the last decades seriously to prepare for the end. The busy and powerful Emperor Charles V abdicated in 1555 and spent the last three years of his life in semi-monastic seclusion. However, in considering the essence of life, death should be accepted as part of the process. One is more able to face the prospect of death after giving up full-time work if some thought has been given to this inevitable end during the years of work and activity. It is important to avoid the pessimism which can characterise old age, to avoid the cynicism which begins to see existence as a gloomy process of walking a road which only has the cemetery gates at its end. Such an attitude can lead either to despair or to a philosophy of "eat, drink and be merry for tomorrow we die". Unfortunately, Somerset Maughan's view that, "Dying is a very dull, dreary affair. And my advice to you is to have nothing whatever to do with it." cannot be sustained indefinitely. Neither attitude is conducive to good living and can lead to unhappiness or a constant regret for lost youth.

Whether one is religious or not, it is crucial that in retirement, thought is given to the deeper vision of existence and the purpose of life. We humans have the unique gift to be able to think about thinking and therefore we have power over the direction of our thoughts and lives. In old age it is important that we give time and thought to these matters. There are books to be read, philosophies to consider and patterns of meditation which can help in facing the vicissitudes of old age and the inevitable fact of death. We must try to make our lives a work of art which is a help and inspiration to those around us. There is much we can do when we give up active employment but we can only be truly effective if we deepen our understanding of the purposes and objects of life. This means being ready to give thought and time to improving our understanding of existence and the way to follow good patterns of living. To put it crudely, it means time to think about religion, ethics and philosophy and not just of golf, bridge and holidays. And to quote Samuel Johnson,

> It matters not how a man dies, but how he lives. The act of dying is not of importance, it lasts so short a time.

PP

Index